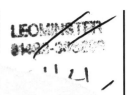

Silent Child

Also by Toni Maguire

Silent Child

A life of fear and a story
of survival

TONI
MAGUIRE

with EMILY SMITH

JOHN BLAKE

Published by John Blake Publishing
An imprint of Bonnier Books UK
80–81 Wimpole St,
Marylebone,
London W1G 9RE

www.bonnierbooks.co.uk

Paperback – 978-1-789-463-05-7
eBook – 978-1-789-463-06-4
Audiobook – 978-1-786-069-93-1

A CIP catalogue of this book is available from the British Library.

Designed by IDSUK (Data Connection) Ltd
Printed and bound in Great Britain by Clays Ltd, Elcograf S.p.A.

1 3 5 7 9 10 8 6 4 2

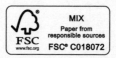

John Blake Publishing is an imprint of
Bonnier Books UK
www.bonnierbooks.co.uk

To my partner and my two amazing girls.

Contents

Part Two

Prologue

Most of us enjoy visiting the past. Sometimes old photo albums are taken out, their contents flicked through. Then, with fingers pointing to the pictures that have caught our attention, we reminisce and chuckle about the times in our lives that they depict. Other times, we catch the eye of a partner or an old friend when an image leaps out of our memory banks and we find ourselves almost saying in unison, 'Oh, do you remember when—?'

Unlike those happy people with their carefree previous lives, I had packed away my past nearly 15 years earlier. Oh, not into a memory box, more like an illusionary filing cabinet where each drawer is neatly labelled. There were the ones showing the happy times I had spent with my mother's family, labelled 'Look At', while others said 'Leave Well Alone'. So, where are the ones of me before I met my partner, which should be stored safely away in albums? All too often the ones I have been asked to dig out.

Well, apart from a couple taken with my grandmother, which she slid into my hand the last time I visited, I never did have any photographs of those times. There are not in my possession any old albums full of square prints showing the various stages of my development from bouncing, gummy baby to self-conscious teenager.

'They got lost when I moved,' I announce breezily, though this is not true.

Those pictures were just never taken.

* * *

But, today, and no doubt again tomorrow, the wrong drawers of that cabinet will fly open, releasing images I do not wish to see. For they have been busy visiting me since they managed to escape. They float behind my closed eyes, sneak into my dreams, even interrupt the odd quiet moment I try and grab during the daytime. So, what has happened for them to be able to do that?

Well, a small person has managed, in no particular order, to open those drawers. The ones I had so firmly slammed shut when I escaped the place I had been forced to call home. How I wish, when they come into my mind, I could remain selective as to the ones I agree to look at. For I still want to hold on to those happy times spent with my mother's family right up until the age of five. But no, each time I try and look at them, the others push them aside triumphantly to show me their darkness. Oh, if only I could erase those sections of my past. But despite all my efforts, it's something I have failed to do.

Another memory, one that is neutral – a voice – entered my head not so long ago. It came from a teacher who had given me a gold star for an essay. 'It's good, Emily,' she was telling me with a warm smile, 'just be careful when you write a story to always start at the beginning.' But then many books start at the end and travel back in time so I'm not finding that to be a binding method.

Well, in my case, without the part of my story that is unfolding daily, I might well have succeeded in keeping all the drawers locked. And then there would be nothing to tell, would there? So, what caused those drawers to fly open, releasing all those images, you might ask. I mean, who was responsible for that?

Why, none other than my daughter, my mini-me.

* * *

It's now over 15 years since I spent Christmas in the House of Horrors, yet I still struggle at this time of the year. I'm on edge the whole time – something will go wrong, my partner will get mad at me, like he can when guests are expected – those are my thoughts the whole time. And then comes the big clean-up before his dad gets here . . . *Hello, silent panic attacks, my old friend.* I'm messy, that's no big news, and the whole bathroom clean-up reminds me of my stepdad's rages. Every slap, every pulling of the hair, name calling, every tear shed . . . they all come back to haunt me like a slap in the face.

You know things were bad when you're not religious yet prayed to a god you didn't believe in to make it all stop. I tried one year as an 11-year-old to drink my pain away. Luckily enough, we didn't have much alcohol in the house so I picked a bottle of Bacardi. The smell alone made me almost throw up. More than likely, this saved me from alcoholism. That, and the constant fear he would know and beat me again.

I'm back to today, this day I so desperately want to enjoy and be present for my daughters. But I can't silence the voice inside, saying I'm messing the whole thing up.

The kids are mostly happy, I think – at least, I hope so. Getting away from France and them is only the start. Quieting their voices, and not being the little girl with all her fears I once was, is the hardest part. You think once you leave, it'll be OK. Now it'll all be great, there'll be no reason to feel afraid or depressed – after all, you survived hell. What could be worse, right? But you can never escape the ghosts from the past, they live forever in your head.

Part One

Chapter 1

On those rare occasions when two-year-old Isabelle is fast asleep and five-year-old Sonia plays contentedly with her toys, I sink gratefully into a chair, a cup of tea in hand.

Well, what mother doesn't seize every opportunity to do the same?

That's not always to say that I find the time restful. All too often watching my daughter neatly line up each object in her toy box or rearrange her dolls to be in the exact position she wants takes me down the path leading to my own childhood. A path I have tried my hardest not to tread. I have come to understand why this happens: it is because she is just such a small version of me. At least, that's what her father said the first time he held her. One look at her tiny face, her long limbs and fuzz of dark blonde hair, and with a beam of absolute joy he said, 'She's a tiny you, Emily.' What I didn't know then was just how much of a version of me she was going to turn into. Not that I gave my partner Patrick's remark much attention then, I was too focused on my new daughter. The moment I heard that cry as she took her first breath, a wave of intense, pure love washed over me. And when the nurse laid her on my breast, my arms rose instinctively to hold her.

'She's perfect,' I murmured, 'just perfect.' The second thought that ran through my head as I cradled her was that I would always protect her. 'You will have a happy childhood,' I whispered to her as I vowed silently to make sure of that.

During those first few days when I arrived home from the hospital, Patrick's mother, Irene, was there to help. 'You need to rest a little,' she told me after she persuaded me to lay my daughter down in her cot. The moment Sonia left me, my arms felt both weightless and empty. If I could, I would have held her against me the whole day. Instead, I lay on my side, one hand brushing the edge of her cot while I listened to the music of her breathing. I simply loved the sounds she made, that quick inhalation of breath she took before pushing it out fast. Hearing those tiny, shallow baby breaths moved me almost to tears.

I remember so clearly the first time I noticed her eyes were following me, and later, how she kicked out her legs that had grown plump and firm. Then there was the day she smiled up at me. And no, I was certain it was not wind, no matter what the health visitor told me! Oh, there's not a day of her development that is not firmly etched in my mind.

It took over two years before I spotted the signs that told me she was much more of a small replica of me than Patrick or I had first thought. It began when she started eating the same solid food as us. My hand was pushed aside the first time I tried to feed her the same way I had fed her the pureed food of just one colour: right from the start, she wanted her own spoon. And then I realised why.

However difficult she found it at first, she busied herself grouping each vegetable together carefully. Mashed potato must not touch a carrot, the carrot must be separate from the pea.

The first time we saw the determined expression on her face as, wielding her spoon, she made sure the food on her plate was arranged to her liking, my partner's sparkling green eyes crinkled with amusement as they met mine.

'Told you she was a mini-you, didn't I?'

Yes, she certainly was, I realised. But then with all the time we spent together, I suppose I was her role model, wasn't I?

'She's just copying me,' I said, then burst out laughing when I gazed down at my plate with its same neat arrangement of vegetables.

But there were other signs, weren't there, other than her fussiness with food? Ones she could not have copied. Signs that showed she had inherited even more of my childhood idiosyncrasies, such as the screams when I brushed her hair. Over the months it had grown from easy-to-look-after fine baby fuzz to thick curls.

You most probably just pulled it too hard, I told myself at first, rushing to the shops to buy a gallon or two of detangling serum. Well, that helped, even if I now spent half an hour or so brushing carefully, a small section at a time. So, that was not too bad.

But her baths, now, they were *really* hard.

From the first day Sonia was lifted gently into the family bath to the accompaniment of ear-piercing wails and flaying limbs, she expressed just how much she hated it, especially when her hair was washed and rinsed using the shower attachment. Not only that, she screamed if a drop of water clung to an eyelash and shuddered when shampoo was rubbed into her scalp or baby lotion onto her body.

It was that first time when we progressed from baby bath to the family bath, my arms holding her while Sonia's screams rocketed around the room, that a memory was unleashed that I had locked away all those years ago. Just for a split second, instead of seeing my hands on my daughter's shoulders, another pair, much larger than mine, with a smattering of coarse black hair on their backs, appeared. And suddenly it was not my daughter who was in front of me but my terrified younger self. Knowing what was about to happen, she was trying frantically to wriggle away from those hands. She could hear the mocking gleeful laughter ringing in her ears as like a thousand stinging hailstones, water gushed down from the shower.

I could remember clearly what happened next and how my five-year-old self had screamed and sobbed. I could almost feel the rawness in her throat as, still dripping with water, she tried to stand, only to find her legs were too weak as though there were no longer any supporting bones beneath the flesh. She collapsed then, five-year-old me, gasping for air as she struggled to breathe.

Sonia, I vowed to myself, *I will never let anything like that happen to you. I will always make your bathtimes safe.*

From that day on, I think of everything I can to make bathtime a fun time. I tell her jokes, I make up games like running her rubber duck up and down the water and float little plastic toys, though there are minimal results there. In fact, the only thing that works is making as many funny faces as I can, something she finds simply hilarious.

'More!', then 'More, Mummy!' become her catchphrases as soon as she adds a few more words to her vocabulary, and by the time I lift her out of the bath, my whole face aches. But at least there have been a few giggles, even the odd snorting little laugh, which are a lot easier on the ears than those early piercing screams. But all this did not stop the one question that was worrying me from entering my head continuously. The one I asked the health visitor about repeatedly from the moment my daughter turned two.

'How can you explain the fact that she's still not really talking?'

Each time she went to great lengths to reassure me that my daughter was healthy and clearly bright.

'Well, children develop at different stages. She's advanced in everything else. I mean, she was potty-trained before she was one, wasn't she? And just look at those drawings, they look like the work of an older child now, don't they?' she said in her calm and soothing voice.

That was all true, but the niggling worry stayed in my head. A worry I did my best to ignore for another year. I knew she was as bright as a button so why couldn't I content myself with that? Hadn't I glowed with pride when she was given educational toys that were part puzzles and after a quick scrutiny worked them out at twice the speed of an average three-year-old? So, I tried out another one where the packaging informed me it was 'suitable for four- to six-year-olds'.

The same result.

But that niggle of worry still refused to go away. Sonia might be as like me as it was possible to be except I could speak at three. I remember that all right – it was my ability to talk that got me in so much trouble. Another memory of my childhood that, not wishing to see, I pushed aside, only to find for once it was replaced with one that made me smile.

Me, somewhere between three and four, curled up on the rug in my grandmother's house, a bowl of chocolate ice cream on my lap. I'd stopped stuffing it in my mouth to say something. I can't remember what, just that she was laughing at whatever it was I had told her.

'Such a little chatterbox you are, Emily,' she said with a beaming smile.

So, I could speak well then, couldn't I?

I had to accept that each day it was becoming increasingly obvious that Sonia's speech was noticeably behind what was expected for her age group. Not just slower than mine had been, but slower than all the other three-year-olds in her nursery. Not only that, but when she learnt a new word she liked the sound of, she would hold it in her mouth so she could repeat it over and over again. That was when I brought in a speech therapist. But I heard the same comforting words coming from her as I had from the health visitor: 'She's bright, children develop at different paces.'

Reassurances I forced myself to believe.

'Her speech is improving,' said the speech therapist after a few weeks. 'Stop worrying, she's a healthy, clever little girl.'

Maybe she should have told me what her real thoughts were then. Or perhaps she believed I knew the answers to those questions I never asked.

There's nothing like parental denial, is there? So, I chose to believe everything would sort itself out.

When Sonia was strong enough to hold my hand as we walked, she pulled on it hard as she hopped across the pavement's white lines. She had refused to walk on them since she had taken her first steps, but then, I told myself, so did I. And as for a white kerb . . . well, I stepped over it quickly enough too, didn't I? It must have been seeing my movements that made her little body stiffen in concentration before she leapt over it. Each time she succeeded, her wide, triumphant smile told me what she was thinking: that we had both escaped something bad happening to us. How did I know that? Because that was what I had also thought when I was her age. Not that I ever worked out what exactly the bad thing would be. But then I had good reason to feel continuous fear whereas there was nothing in her life to cause her to be afraid.

She just thinks we're playing a game, I told myself then. Deep down, didn't I really know this was not the case?

It was not until the day when we decided to picnic on the beach that I finally began to face up to the fact that I needed to talk to a professional, someone more senior than my health visitor and speech therapist. Not to friends or my partner's family, who just wanted to reassure me that

Sonia was perfect – which of course she was. But there was no getting away from the fact that she was different to other children and it was why she was different that I needed the answers to.

* * *

It was two years ago when we woke to one of those bright, warm, sunny days that all of Ireland welcomes. After one glance out the window at a cloudless sky, Patrick and I decided it was the perfect day for taking a picnic to Barley Cove. It was those beaches and coves that made Patrick long to return to Ireland – it's also the perfect place to bring up children. Because it was a weekend, we knew the cove, with its safe, shallow estuary, would quickly become crowded with young families so we wasted as little time as possible, throwing food and soft drinks plus those important bottles of sun lotion into our chiller bags.

On arrival, we were lucky enough to find a secluded sunny expanse of sand. Blankets and cushions were laid out, a large golf umbrella positioned to give us shade and sun cream rubbed carefully on all three of us. Once done, cold drink in hand, I leant back against a boulder and began to relax while Patrick started building a sandcastle for Sonia.

'Come on, Emily, give us a hand here,' he said as he began to construct a wall from what seemed like a million grains of sand.

'Just a moment,' I replied, glancing at our daughter. 'She looks a bit hot, doesn't she? I'll take her sandals off, she'll be cooler then.' Bending down, I removed them. That was the first summer Sonia could walk unaided and Patrick and I smiled as we watched her take her first hesitant steps on the beach. Smiles that disappeared the second the screaming began.

This was not just crying which I could divert her from. I knew from the way she was standing, mouth wide open, arms flailing the air, it was the start of a full-blown meltdown. I also understood straight away that it was the touch of the sand between her toes that had caused it. Kneeling beside her, telling her everything was going to be all right, I used my fingers to brush it gently away from those tiny gaps between each toe. But no matter how often I repeated this process until every grain of sand was gone, with her face turned up to the sky and her body rigid, she continued screaming.

From the amount of head turning that day, such a scene on that beach was clearly never witnessed before. I just hoped none of the people there had also been in Tesco when Sonia had her previous meltdown. The amount of tutting from women I had heard that day made me want to shout at them. Remembering the glares of disapproval received then and the remarks overheard about bad parenting, I was convinced this time we were minutes away from mobile phones being pulled out, numbers for social services being looked up.

For once, even Patrick looked helpless. Still, he had not been in the supermarket with me that day, nor was he the one who had dealt with Sonia's early outbursts when her hair was shampooed. He had never been present before when she had a public meltdown. All I could do was sit back on my heels and wait for the screaming to stop. Which it finally did once her strength deserted her. With heart-breaking sobs, she sank to the ground. Time stood still, all I was aware of was her distress. Nothing else mattered – not the stares, not my worry, just my daughter as I crouched beside her, whispering all the soothing words I could think of until at last, she was quiet. For a moment I was relieved, thinking it was all over, until, ignoring me, she curled into a tight little ball and, bending over her, I saw her eyes were both vacant and unfocused.

'No, don't touch her,' I told Patrick sharply as he leant down, arms outstretched, ready to scoop her up. Because I knew, didn't I? She had retreated into a sad, lonely place. Everything around her had simply disappeared from her vision and until a feeling of safety was restored, she would not be able to leave it.

I think I must have held my breath. Like my daughter, I was almost oblivious to anything happening around me. I knew at least one woman had approached, offering help – something I left my partner to deal with. I just wanted to take Sonia in my arms, whisper to her that she was already in a safe place, but I understood that day I had to wait for her to return to us in her own time.

It seemed like hours passed before blinking, she sat up and I was able to hold her, but once home, we agreed it had only been just over ten minutes.

Patrick looked wretched.

'I had attacks like that when I was little,' I said haltingly.

'You never told me.'

'No, I managed to control them when I was older and then I just blamed them on what was happening in my life.'

'Well, there's nothing like that happening in hers, is there? Come on, Emily, she might have inherited a lot of you, but not your memories!'

No, there wasn't anything like that. And I had to accept that she had not copied my behaviour this time. OK, I too had always hated the feeling of grass or sand beneath my feet, but not enough to have the reaction my daughter had. I knew then that I had finally run out of all the excuses I used to explain her behaviour. Patrick was right, she was not just copying me. That was the first thing we agreed on. The second was that we needed to see someone in the medical field who specialised in children's behaviour.

'I'll talk to our doctor and I'm certain he will recommend someone suitable,' I said with as much positivity as I could muster.

A plan I put into action the following Monday.

*   *   *

When I blurted out all my concerns to my GP, he looked hardly surprised.

'Yes, it sounds as though she does take after you, Emily. I think now would be a good time to get her professionally assessed.'

Not that he said exactly what she was to be assessed for. He mentioned a clinic, which he assured me was very good, and he would do a referral letter, make the appointment and get back in touch with me.

So that's that, I thought, about to rise to leave. But oh no, he still had a whole barrage of questions for me.

'So, you have an honours degree in English and French,' he said eventually, 'but what about your Maths?'

My mind shot back to being in senior school and the teachers' disbelief as to how I came to my answers.

'Every one of my Maths problems was correct, except I could not write down how I worked out the answers. I mean, numbers just flew into my head. It was as if all on their own they could add, subtract, divide and multiply so fast I could never catch them, an explanation hardly ever believed back then. My teachers were always annoyed with me. They kept saying I must know how I came to the right answer, but I never did really.'

The doctor smiled when I explained that to him as if he completely understood.

'So, you failed Maths not because your answers were wrong, but because you could not explain how you came by them? In layman's terms that means your brain works as fast as a computer and unfortunately the school did not recognise the reasons you gave them, but then the higher end of the autistic spectrum is often not recognised during childhood.'

That was when I came to the realisation that it was no longer my daughter he was showing an interest in. And how I learnt that I was autistic. Now, you would have thought I could have worked that out for myself, wouldn't you? I mean, there's quirky and there's different. But then with all the labels my parents pinned on me with harsh words and threats, being autistic had not been one of them.

* * *

The doctor explained both my and my daughter's fear of the touch of certain things, such as water, grass and sand, was known as sensory processing problems. In other words, to us it was painful, while to others, pleasant or just mildly irritating.

'Luckily,' he added in his reassuring voice, 'schools are now far more aware of how autism should be dealt with than they probably were when you were at school. Nowadays, most teachers have an understanding of the problems it can cause and are specifically trained to deal with them sympathetically.'

'You mean problems like meltdowns?'

'Yes, meltdowns and all the other ones as well.'

'Well, it's a long list! I suppose it's a good thing that I have the same problems as her, only not so extreme, isn't it?'

I could almost read the doctor's mind, saying, *Well, that's one way to look at it*. Instead, he continued to ask me questions.

Questions I wished he would leave well alone.

'Tell me,' he went on, pen poised over my medical notes in front of him, 'how did your mother deal with those problems – like washing your hair, for instance?'

That question caused one of my locked filing cabinet drawers to fly open and there was my mother, hairbrush in hand, a less-than-sympathetic expression on her face, tugging and pulling at my tangles while I screamed out in pain.

'If you don't stop that noise now, I'll shave it all off!' she threatened as she gave my head an impatient thwack with the stiff and sharply bristled brush. Now the one thing you have to know about people with autism is that they find it difficult to lie so it took some effort to look my doctor squarely in the face and say, 'Oh, she just took her time. We managed.'

'And how about the issues with food?'

As if on cue, the moment the word 'food' left his mouth, another drawer labelled 'Unhappy Mealtimes' shot out. There I was, sat on a hard chair, my head only a little higher than the top of the shiny dark wooden table. On the white plate in front of me was a chunk of red meat. I could see the blood oozing from it and knew what would happen if I managed to force a piece into my mouth: I would gag and gag until my throat stung with the burning vomit rushing from my stomach. There were those two voices ringing in my ears: my mother's harsh one, telling me if I dared chuck up my food again, I could clean it up myself and the other, a male one, laughing before he told me to just imagine it was a chocolate ice cream on my plate.

'Then you can swallow every bit down,' he announced mockingly.

There was my young self between a rock and a hard place, having to decide which was worse: eating the disgusting bloodied meat and gagging, or being hit before being sent off to bed.

'Oh, she didn't take much notice, Doctor,' I manage to croak out.

'Mmm . . .' was his only reply as he shot me an appraising look. Something told me he did not believe me.

'And how about school, how was that for you?'

'Good,' I replied. 'I did well in classes and was popular.'

Well, that was not altogether true either, was it?

Chapter 2

If those drawers began opening as I sat with my doctor, they just about hurled themselves at me afterwards – and not in any particular order either. There were times when the reflection that stared back at me from the mirror was not my adult self, but my unhappy younger one when she was the same age as my daughter is now, though with her furrowed brow and tear-filled eyes, there is little resemblance between Sonia's happy smiling face and mine. My younger self's expression showed all too clearly her bewilderment as to why her mother was angry with her most of the time, while her father made no bones about wanting to avoid his small daughter as much as possible. With her lack of self-worth, she believed it was because there was something inherently wrong with her. She was different, wasn't she? The young Emily knew that because her cousins told her repeatedly that she was – she just didn't understand why that was (later, I was to stop being so weird).

It was, I knew, the questions that the doctor had asked about eating that had made that drawer, labelled 'Eating Punishments', spring open. That red meat came into my vision, as did the image of me spewing it up onto the floor.

Once open, my mother's shrill voice echoing down through the years followed me wherever I went: the bedroom, the bathroom, the lounge and even the garden. There was just no escape from hearing the words that had once disturbed me so much – 'Bad, you're bad! I don't know what I've done to deserve being burdened with a child like you. You're disgusting! Don't you sit there thinking I'm going to clear up your mess.' With that, she stomped out of the room to return with a wad of newspaper, a cloth and the pail almost full of very hot soapy water: 'Now, this floor better be clean when I inspect it, do you hear me, Emily?'

Well, I could hardly help but hear her – every word was ringing in my ears. Not that she waited for an answer before she told me to get myself off to bed as soon as I was done there.

I could see her, my younger self, knelt on the floor, cloth in hand, scooping up her own vomit while trying desperately not to be sick again. And then I think of Sonia and how Patrick and I handled her having an upset stomach, only a week earlier. She had caught a nasty bug that was doing the rounds. I had sat her on my knee while I gently stroked her back and then without warning, spurt after spurt of projectile vomiting hit my shoulder, landed on the couch and trickled down her clothes. Her face crumpled with shock and we could see tears were not very far away.

'Oh dear,' I said quickly, 'let's get you cleaned up.'

Between us she was soon consoled, hands and face wiped clean, a new nightdress slipped over her head, and then, still telling her it was not her fault, I cuddled her until her eyes started to close drowsily.

'Come on, sweetheart, time for bed,' I whispered before carrying her into her bedroom.

Two scenes: same subject, no similarity. But then Patrick and I have produced a happy child who knows her parents love and understand her. I made a promise when she was born that she would grow up with the confidence that I myself was denied.

A happy thought entered my head then. It was during the summer of 2017 when Sonia and I were walking on a path and her tugging at my hand made it clear that she desperately wanted to walk not in the middle but right on the edge of the path and I saw that it was a different colour.

'OK,' I said, moving to it, and together, we played a game of staying on the line between the two shades. She shot me the widest smile then, a smile that said, 'You get me, Mum, don't you?'

'Of course I do,' my returning smile and a quick squeeze of her hand told her. As a kid, hadn't I tried to do the exact same thing? On pedestrian crossings I sent my cousin mad when walking to school as I jumped over the dark sections – I only wanted to touch the white markings. Nothing bad would happen to me that day if I did, that was what I would tell myself. Though I rarely managed to succeed for my hand was yanked hard as whichever cousin was lumbered hissed at me to stop acting strangely.

Strange it might be, but I still have those thoughts – that's OCD for you.

Chapter 3

It is those comparisons that allow my sneaky inner voice to pester me with questions. *What would you have been like now, had you been cared for like Sonia is? Would you have had those fears that won't go away? And the nightmares that wake you up in a cold sweat, when behind your lids you either almost walk over a cliff or find yourself a prisoner in a room without windows or doors? Would they have even visited you? Wouldn't you instead have shut your eyes and drifted off into a dreamless, blank space?*

And then that voice tells me to get a grip. To stop blaming myself for being the reason my father turned away each time I tried to get his attention. *All right*, the voice says, *he knew you were different and didn't like it, but as he was an adult and you were only a child, who really was to blame? Well, it wasn't you, was it?*

And what about your mother, do you still think her cruelty was your fault? That woman who used words like a bayonet, jabbing and jabbing until she was satisfied that she had sufficiently hurt you?

And here's the question you have to deal with: do you believe that if none of that had happened, you would have been a different person? The answer to that, I'm sure, is yes. Wouldn't I have been the confident student, the confident young woman and the confident mother I have pretended to the world that I am?

Angry with myself for allowing negativity to enter my mind, I push aside the waves of sadness that threaten to engulf me almost as quickly as those questions came into my head. *For God's sake, Emily, count your blessings, why don't you? Think of the present and the future and don't dwell on the past. Now is the time to take charge. Open up those drawers yourself, one at a time. Deal with what's inside them and, once done, put them away again. After all, you have two little girls who need you. Not to mention a partner who has accepted everything about you, so just confront your past and deal with it. Because if you don't, as your daughter grows, you will keep seeing yourself at her age. And then what will happen? Those drawers will keep flying open and you'll be a mess. And that's no good for anyone now, is it?*

How I wished that voice would just shut up, but then we never want to listen to the truth about ourselves, do we?

And will they stay closed then?

If you have dealt with them, they will.

So, open the one labelled 'My Mother's Family Before Him' first. What's inside there is happy, isn't it?

Chapter 4

Before you meet *him* in my pages, I am going to introduce the family I used to have. Because I want you to see them as I did, then you will understand what it was that I lost.

* * *

Of course, the very beginning of my story is not fixed firmly in my mind, but over the years some memories have managed to resurface, others I put together from scraps of conversation I managed to overhear.

My parents' home was in an area where wages were low and the crime rate was high. Despite that, up until I was five, I saw that world as a friendly place. Not even when my mother and I moved to another flat in an even poorer area, where every weekend the wails of police sirens filled the air, did I change my mind. In fact, I took very little notice of my surroundings there, mainly because most of my time was spent with Mum's family. There was my widowed grandmother, a short, plump figure, with dark hair turning grey and those large blue eyes that I have inherited, my two aunts, Lizzy and Maria, who were younger versions of their mother, a couple of uncles and an assortment of cousins of both sexes and all ages. Apart from my parents, I was surrounded by people who loved me and I in turn adored them.

So, for the most part I was not aware of the arrests of local drug dealers and petty thieves, nor did I take much notice of the shouts and screams that usually accompanied them. They were just part of the familiar background I had grown used to. In fact, right up until I began school and my mother brought *him* home, there was nothing much for me to worry about.

My mother's large family was well known in our small village. My eldest cousin was a great football player and my uncle was the local policeman. They were the kind of family no one had a bad word to say about – well, apart from my father, of course. He was quite a different matter, my little eavesdropping ears discovered.

While I was both happy and content when I was with my aunts and grandmother, my memories of being with my mother are very different. Unlike my aunts and grandmother, Mum was a bony woman, all sharp edges and a face that seldom broke into a smile. Well, certainly not in my direction anyhow. With her fair hair and clever use of make-up, there was no doubt that she was attractive – well, I had heard her sisters saying that. I still wish I had just one memory of her picking me up, giving me a cuddle or even playing with me, but there isn't one. Then, maybe that's not so surprising when I was the one deemed responsible for breaking up her marriage.

At least that's what my parents told me.

Not that I have a really good picture of what exactly I did to cause it. That information I gleaned over the years from both my parents as well as listening to my aunts' gossip. The excuse that I had not even turned five at the time is not one that carried any weight – for years I carried the blame for that deed. So, it was lucky for me that my main carers during those vital formative years were my aunts and grandmother, a trio of dark-haired, blue-eyed women who thought I could do no wrong. And how I loved them! It was their soft arms that picked me up when I fell. Scraped knees were gently cleaned and sweets 'to make everything better' popped in my mouth. Before I was put to bed in the evenings, the aunts and my grandmother took turns in cuddling me against their comfortable, rounded bodies when they introduced me to various characters living in books. Now, years later, I can still hear their gentle voices telling me I was special.

Weekends were simply the best times to spend with the family. Free from school, my host of cousins and their friends were there for me to play with. Even the children who were only slightly older than me had been told it was their job to protect me. Not only that, I must not be teased for those little idiosyncrasies that were becoming more noticeable. The twisting of my hair and the sucking of my tongue when agitated were the two most obvious mannerisms although there were others too.

Now, how would I know that?

My mother screamed it out at me. Told me my cousins thought I was peculiar. And did I really think they wanted to play with me? Well, they didn't, they were only obeying their parents.

Trust Mum's voice to get in my head and spoil those good memories.

I can remember the day she told me that; my grandmother had made me a dress – raspberry pink, with a square neck – and Aunt Lizzy had just sewn up a pink cardigan she had been knitting for me. When my mother came to collect me and I showed them to her, her mouth tightened in a thin line: 'They spoil you,' she hissed as soon as we were out of earshot.

It was once we were back at our flat that the rest of her venom spilled out.

Don't let that part in, my voice told me, making me relegate it to the drawer labelled 'Mother's Insults' and slam it shut. *Now, go back to those happy days you spent with your grandmother.* Obediently, I take myself back in time until I am in Gran's kitchen, inhaling the various aromas of her cooking. I am listening to the trio as they gossip about Saturday's family gathering and who's going to be cooking what. Even now those memories can still bring a smile to my face.

On Saturdays, as soon as spring arrived, my grandmother and I would make our way to where my aunts lived. She would help me dress in my dark blue dungarees and red T-shirt before checking in the mirror that her hair was tidy and putting on her lipstick. Then, picking up her handbag, she would say each time, 'Ready, are you?' and open the door. Once we were outside her tall terraced house with its bow-fronted windows and rooms full of dark furniture, ornaments and gilt-framed family photos, she would take my hand as we walked the short distance to where the rest of her family lived.

Both my uncles and their wives lived at the same address. Not in the same house, but on the same plot of land, where they had built their large family homes. There were tall wooden gates that opened onto a gravel driveway leading past the velvety green lawns to the front doors of the adjacent houses.

The moment grey clouds were chased away by a light breeze and a few rays of sun appeared, the families would gather for those homes had certainly been designed for family parties. At the rear of the houses actually joining them together was wooden decking with rattan chairs and sofas covered with plump, brightly coloured cushions and a long wooden table that took up most of the central space. Several feet away from the decking stood the red-bricked built-in barbecue. My aunts busied themselves in the kitchen while my cousins and I were allocated various tasks depending on our ages. Mine was putting out the cushions. The rest carried out drinks, salads and platters of marinated raw meat until the table was practically groaning under the weight.

That meat, all pink and glistening, was something I avoided looking at. Just one glimpse made my fingers tighten round my hair as I pulled it hard, the sharp pain calming me momentarily. The uncles, both rather portly men with thick, dark hair and wide, white smiles, always made it clear that they were the ones in charge of the outside grill. I had heard my aunts say, with affectionate chuckles, that they rarely lifted a finger in the house though. Outside was clearly a different matter – they took over both the lighting of the barbecue and the grilling of the meat with enthusiasm. Once the embers were just glowing red, with beers in one hand and large forks in the other, they would turn the meat until it was cooked as they said 'to perfection', before being heaped onto plates.

'You would think they had hunted that meat themselves, wouldn't you, instead of us getting it from the butcher and tenderising it!' the aunts would joke each time, while I tried to block my nose from inhaling what was for me the nauseous smell of meat. Not my favourite smell, though winding my hair around my fingers helped take my mind off it.

Seeing my fingers busy in my hair, my grandmother would lean over, take my hand gently in hers and whisper reassuringly that there was different food for me. Usually it was chicken and sweetcorn. She knew not only of my dislike of any sign of blood on my plate, but of my need to have the vegetables sorted into different colours. To avoid that problem at these family events, she made sure there was only one vegetable for me every time. She never said anything about it, neither did she mention my twisting and pulling my hair – I think she sensed it was something I did when stressed and just accepted it.

Once the meal was eaten, my cousins and I would help stack the dishes before running off into the large garden to play games. Kicking a ball into the net was one of the most popular ones. Ben, my favourite cousin, who was several years older than me, would grab hold of my hand and pull me out of my seat. Not that he had to force me; he was the cousin who, with his floppy blond hair and sun-tanned, lithe body, I totally idolised.

'Come on, Sprat! Let's kick a ball around,' he would say laughingly. Surprisingly, even though I was the smallest of the lot, aiming the ball correctly and shooting it through the goal posts was something I was good at.

'Well done,' he would tell me, giving me a high five each time the ball shot through them, 'you're going to be the next great footballer in our family one day!'

I would glow with pride at this praise.

Yes, my memories of being in that garden with my cousins are happy ones – I felt safe there.

Sometimes my parents made an appearance at these gatherings. My father always looked slightly uneasy as he tried to make conversation with the uncles, while Mum chatted to her sisters, the aunts. Usually the excuse that it took them time to get back to where we lived was made and so we left long before anyone else. It was then that I would hold my breath, hoping that I would be allowed to stay another night with Gran.

Luckily for me, my mother often used the excuse that as our family home was not within walking distance, it might be better if I stayed over. If she did not say it first, my grandmother would suggest: 'It's a bit of a walk for her, why don't I get someone to run her back tomorrow?' Usually, Mum would agree.

It was true my parents did live much further away but there were buses, weren't there? I guess there was more than one reason why they made their excuses to leave early and were happy for me to remain there. First, it gave them another day without me and what must surely be my irritating habits and second, Dad felt that he was just tolerated, which is not the same as being welcomed, by my mother's family. Not that I knew then that my father's father had 'done time'. Again, my little ears had heard that expression used more than once. So perhaps being in the company of his policeman brother-in-law, who had been part of the team who arrested his father long before Dad met Mum, was hardly enjoyable.

Whatever the reason, being with the family was best for me. In their homes I was never shouted at, ordered to leave the room or told that I was making anyone feel sick listening to me. No, there I felt totally loved. The few photos I have managed to salvage from that time show a little blue-eyed, blonde girl, tall for her age, smiling happily into the camera lens. In fact, the only two people who did not seem besotted by me were my own parents.

Chapter 5

If my grandmother saw only good things about me, she also saw my mother in a rosy light that she hardly deserved. Everything was my father's fault, not hers – not necessarily an opinion completely shared by the aunts, her sisters, even though they had little time for him.

More than once I had overheard them saying that he might be good-looking and have a certain amount of charm, but he was also uncouth – a word I took to my cousin Ben to ask what it meant before adding it to my growing vocabulary. 'A bit rough' was his answer. By the grin on his face, I guess he knew where I had heard it and who they had been talking about. Knowing what Mum's family really thought of Dad did not stop me seeking his approval though. Unlike my mother, he never shouted at me or told me to get lost. Instead, he would turn away and look at anything in the room apart from his daughter.

But I was not the only one who was aware of my parents' lack of interest in me. I overheard comments made by the three female relatives when they thought I was out of earshot. They seemed to have forgotten that small children can just about hear grass grow, but then they were a trio whose hobby was gossiping.

The moment I heard my parents' names mentioned my ears were on full alert. I mean, maybe we are always more curious about those people who do not love us than the ones who do. I know we would have to go back to the beginning of that marriage to get a full idea of the family dynamics. Not that I can for there was never much said about how my mum and dad met, or how long they had been together before I arrived. It was the present my aunts and grandmother talked about, with much sighing and concerns about me.

'He was never right for her,' my grandmother said more than once.

And working in the same place hardly helped, they all agreed.

'Not good, that,' said Aunt Lizzy. 'Couples never do well when they spend all their time together.'

'Get to know each other too well, you mean,' sniffed her sister, Maria.

So that was the first bit of knowledge that was stored in my mind. The second bit they would certainly not have wanted me to hear, but then children lying on a couch with their eyes closed are not always asleep.

'I mean,' said one of the aunts, 'spending all that time together must have been what put those cracks in their marriage. Oh, the rows they had! And didn't we have to listen for hours about how bad he was to her? But did they sit down and try and work something out, or let's face it, decide it was over?'

'No, not her,' my other aunt replied with a snort of contempt. 'She never did like the word "Miss" in front of her name so what did they do instead? They had a save-the-relationship baby. Hadn't given a thought to the reality that babies cry, need feeding, changing and bathing. Oh no, they thought that would make everything all right between them.'

Suddenly, I understood from the glances in my direction which I could see beneath half-closed eyes that it was me they were talking about.

It was me who was the save-the-relationship baby!

A bit ironic, that.

Chapter 6

Not that my parents' marriage crumbled overnight. My dad had other ways of occupying his time, which must have provided him with a defence against Mum's nagging. Now, it was clear that neither she nor her sisters had any idea that he had started cheating on her. Perhaps everyone in our family thought that it was his wife who put the happy expression on his face – if they did, they got that wrong. Something they would have found out, had they been able to make themselves invisible before creeping into their home and listening to just how my parents spoke to each other.

That idea would have flown straight out of their heads then.

In many ways, as small children can, I was able to do just that. For angry adults rarely realise just how much they are listened to. When I stayed with my grandmother, crayoning away busily, both she and my aunts appeared to believed that particular activity blocked my ears and prevented me from hearing. Over the time I spent with them, through titbits of their conversations, I learnt that none of my mother's family considered my father was good enough for her – a heartfelt belief that they had no problem discussing. Listening to them, I discovered he was in a badly paid job and that was why my poor mother had to go out to work. On top of that, he was content to live in an area so rough it was embarrassing, and of course they worried about me.

'I mean,' said Aunt Lizzy, 'just what sort of children is Emily going to mix with on that estate?'

Even so, I understood that while they might not approve of my mother's choice of husband, they hoped, more for my sake than hers, that the cracks in my parents' marriage had now been filled in and peace was reigning. That might well have been the case had it not been for one thing: my loose-lipped mouth. Well, those were the words my dad, red-faced with anger, shouted at me when he discovered that I was the one responsible for letting my mother know just what he was up to. Though looking back, I think maybe as I was not quite five and he was an adult, perhaps he should have been held accountable for his misdeeds.

Whoever was to blame, once my mother's suspicions were confirmed, it was not a good time in our home. She had to face up to the fact that her husband's philandering had been going on for longer than she had already guessed. To make matters worse, who was it he had chosen to have that final extramarital fling with? Why, none other than her best friend, Lily. If that wasn't bad enough, she also worked in the same place as Mum and Dad. In fact, to add insult to injury, it was my mother who had got her the job. All this I learnt through the screams and shouts vibrating through our house.

As an adult, I can just imagine the tension that affair caused between Dad and his girlfriend once it got under way. But then certain types of people get a kick from taking risks and if that was the case, those two must have been on a permanent high. Not that when the affair was brought out into the daylight Lily didn't do the decent thing and disappear from both my father's life and their workplace. Although, when huddled in my bed shivering, I heard enough to know that was not something he wanted. As I listened wretchedly to my mother alternating between sobs and screams of anguish and anger, my father made it pretty clear that if he had to choose one of them, it was not going to be her – a decision that was to change all of our lives, but mine more than theirs. And not for the better either.

In one day my mother lost her husband and the only woman friend she had trusted. Though maybe she should have guessed that with her wide smile and loud laugh, Lily was not what you might call a 'woman's woman'.

The last time I saw her, apart from a certain hardness around her eyes and mouth, she was little changed from when she was young. Thanks, no doubt, I thought uncharitably to generous helpings of Botox and a good hairdresser. When I allow myself to conjure her image up, I always see her as she looked when we first met. Glossy dark hair, shimmering down to her shoulders, olive skin and brown eyes fringed with thick lashes, gazing up at my father. That was when she believed that I was incapable of noticing anything. Another memory skittles into my mind of her hand with its long red-painted nails resting on my mother's arm as they laughed loudly at one of their shared jokes.

Looking back, I would say then that she resembled those models seen on travel brochures advertising warm Mediterranean holidays. 'She's Italian,' my mother had told me when I asked where she came from, 'that's why she always looks so well turned out.' She was still in thrall of Lily's glamour. Gran, on the other hand, with a sniff of disapproval called it 'dressed to the nines', which soon became 'sluttish' when it all blew up. Certainly, there was no doubt that Lily, with her bright red lipstick, high heels and pretty, clinging dresses, always made an effort: 'And she doesn't dress up like that to impress her girlfriends, now does she? Though women like that seldom have any,' my grandmother added, her tone of voice implying Mum should have guessed who it was after Lily began visiting our home.

I can't remember much of what Lily chatted about when she visited apart from that she was only passing on the way to meet friends. No doubt that was her excuse for having doused herself in a sickly-sweet perfume and putting even more of an effort into her appearance. I was too young then to wonder why my mother and Lily were such good friends for they were certainly complete opposites. In those days Mum did not layer on the make-up or wear revealing clothes.

On the odd afternoon when I was with her at the factory, I would watch the two of them on their tea breaks, chatting away. There they would sit, two grown women, giggling like kids at something they both spotted in a magazine, or indulging in a little gossip about some of the people who worked there. I noticed the other women giving her suspicious looks, not that they dented Lily's confidence. She would just whisper something in Mum's ear, which judging by the expressions on their faces was hardly complimentary. Occasionally, her son Paul was also permitted to be with her. 'My mother could not look after him today,' was her excuse. 'Hospital appointment,' she would add in a lowered voice, with a worried crease between her brows when she blagged the foreman.

'All right, just this once,' was always the answer.

I suppose my being allowed the odd visit had to do with both my parents working there. There was never any mention of Lily having a husband or if there ever had been one, a question I had heard muttered from a couple of her workmates. Not that I was interested, I was just pleased that I had found a new playmate near my age to keep me company. Fairly soon after she became friends with Mum, Lily was accepted into our family. It had not taken her long to inveigle invitations to our family parties for herself and Paul. Being a large family, one more child around was barely noticed so he just got treated as an extra cousin. This certainly suited Lily because now whichever relative was babysitting me would happily allow her to leave her son there as well.

Chapter 7

The one thing I can honestly say about myself is that for a long time I was a trusting child. Grown-ups know best, my mother told me repeatedly, so I believed her. Which also means that my child's instinct did not ring any warning bells when Lily began dropping into our house. But let's just say that trust diminished rather on that last Saturday when my father was given the task of keeping an eye on me.

Every few weeks in my mother's family, husbands were placed on child-sitting duties while the three sisters went shopping, before, more importantly, meeting up for lunch. That fateful Saturday, Mum had told Dad and I on the way out that Lily was coming round with Paul: 'We thought Emily and he could play together and you would be free to watch your sports programme,' was all she said, shooting out the door before he could voice any objection.

So, believe it or not, it was she who fixed that I was being left with two people who thought their secret was safe. And before the day was out, the third person in the triangle was to find out the truth of what exactly had been going on for weeks under her very nose. The story, which has been repeated more than once, goes that I caught them at it in the bedroom while they were meant to be watching both me and her son. Just as well I only have a dim memory of that! I know what happened, though.

Remember when I said I was trusting, that I believed what adults told me? That I never questioned them? Well, that was my mistake because the lie my father told me that day was that there were books in the bedroom he wanted to show Lily and I must be good and not disturb them.

Now I knew there were no books in the bedroom, but that didn't stop me believing him. This is why I didn't realise the true meaning of why they were in the bedroom when I shared his feeble excuse with Mum – I just know that when the words came out of my mouth, it was me she shook hard. That was my first lesson in life: the messenger always gets shot.

Dad and Lily must have been looking at books for a long time, I had thought, and I was hungry and so was Paul, but we were too small to reach the biscuits on the shelves above our heads. I stretched and stretched, but it was no use. It was Paul who dared me to go into them. He used words like 'scaredy-cat', which made me take my courage in both hands, open the bedroom door and walk in. My mind's a blur as to what happened next. Paul, who had allowed me as far as the doorway, told me much later that the pair of them pulled the sheets up to their chins and yelled at me to get out. I do remember though how soon after Lily flew from the room, shooting me venomous looks.

'Creepy little sneak!' she spat out, before grabbing her son by the arm and storming out. As she did so, Paul looked at me helplessly.

Now if they hadn't shouted so loudly and made me run from the room crying, I might not have thought to say anything. It all came out a bit later though when my mother noticed the tear streaks on my face.

'What have you been crying about now, Emily?' she asked, giving me one of her impatient shakes.

So, I told her. And there you have it: two people yelling insults at each other, one who blamed a kid's big mouth.

Yes, I really had made a good job of failing in the role of relationship-fixer baby.

Chapter 8

I'm pretty sure now that before that double betrayal there had been other dalliances that had been ignored. But not this one; her husband sleeping with her best friend was not something my mother was going to turn a blind eye to. Very few wives would. And Mum certainly had no intention of it, especially when two young children were the only witnesses to the treachery. While I stood there shaking, I listened to the shouting and heard expressions that I had never heard before, 'your dirty whore' being one that remains fixed in my mind.

Oh, he tried to say I had made it up, that Lily had been gone for ages and that he was in the bedroom on his own. None of which my mother believed.

'She's not clever enough to lie,' was all she said.

Another black mark for me.

'There, I hope you're satisfied,' was all Dad said to me then, and feeling more tears starting up again, I shot into my bedroom as they screamed and shouted at each other some more. The row continued into the small hours until I heard the front door slam and my mother screaming, 'Go on, go to your whore then!'

And that, I learnt the next day, was exactly what he did.

* * *

It only took until the following morning for Mum to realise just what the consequences of her husband's departure were going to mean: primarily, no money coming in. She must have woken up thinking about it for no sooner did she come down the stairs than she was on the phone. I couldn't help but hear her shrill voice barely pausing for breath as she unburdened her woes, first into her mother's ears and then on additional calls to both of her sisters. I guessed breakfast was not on the agenda and wondered what was going to happen next.

I did not have long to wait.

'We're going to Gran's,' she told me, before dashing into her room.

Following her, I saw that all the bedding in my parents' room was scattered over the floor. She must have pulled it off before she had been able to face sleeping in the same bed that, just a few hours earlier, her husband and her so-called friend had sullied. She helped me get dressed before getting ready herself, then it was a quick cup of tea for her, a glass of milk for me and we were off.

Once at Gran's, I saw that my aunts, their eyes wide with curiosity, were already sitting around the kitchen table.

Nothing like their sister almost finding her fickle husband in bed with her best friend to get them running down to Gran's house to hear the story again first-hand.

Almost the moment we walked into the kitchen, the tears started. Tissues appeared as though by magic, and once a wad of them was in one hand and a cup of tea in the other, my mother recounted everything that had happened for the fourth time that morning. Well, not quite *everything* – she downplayed the screaming row that must have kept the whole road awake until the early hours.

I saw the aunts' eyes open even wider when she told them how it was me who had let the cat out of the bag.

'Books in the bedroom, I ask you! What were they thinking? I suppose he thought Emily would believe anything he told her.'

That said just about everything about my parents' level of reading.

'And the worst thing,' she added, 'is that I can't even go into the factory. I mean, how could I work alongside them both again? Can you imagine having to look at that whore with her smug face, cosying up to my lying husband every day?'

Clearly, they couldn't, though that did not stop them all agreeing with her vehemently.

'He will have to pay you maintenance though, won't he?' said Aunt Maria.

'And give you money for Emily as well,' Aunt Lizzy added.

'And just how do I make him do that? He's tight as a tick that one . . .'

'Be sensible, Betty,' said Gran, 'there are laws to protect you. Tom might be devious but he's not stupid, he knows he will have to pay for his daughter so the first thing you need to do is get a solicitor to sort everything out. They will tell him how much child support he will be liable for. And he knows what would happen if he doesn't comply – he'll be in court pretty sharpish. No doubt the judge would insist on an attachment placed on his earnings. Doubt he'd want the company to see that.'

'Attached to what, his measly little pay-packet? He hardly brings home what I would call a decent wage, does he? That's why I had to work. And let's face it, Mum, you can't get blood out of a stone now, can you? Goodness knows what we're going to live on now.'

More sniffs, and more tissues were passed around.

For once it was she and not me who was the centre of attention. In between gasps of disgust, shoulders were squeezed, her back rubbed, even more tea poured. Before she launched yet again into her version of the facts, Gran put her arm around me.

'Let's get you some breakfast,' she said gently and led me out of the kitchen and into her comfortable sitting room. She told me that as a treat I could have my breakfast in there while I watched my favourite video, *Sooty & Co.* 'You'd like that, wouldn't you, darling?' she asked and I nodded a yes.

I think I would have been content to sit with nothing in front of me – anything to get away from the conversation in that kitchen.

Gran must have known that I had heard everything that happened in the house and that my mother had done very little to stop me being caught up in it. Not that she asked any questions. Instead, she just put the video on for me before going back in the kitchen. A few minutes later, she returned with my dish of scrambled eggs, toast and juice on a tray, which she placed on my lap. Seeing I was apparently already absorbed in the video, she patted me on the shoulder and returned to the hub of the house – her kitchen, where the family pow wows always seemed to take place.

All I could think, while I watched Sooty's funny antics, was that I didn't want to go home – I wanted to stay at Gran's, where there was no more shouting and no more tears or blame placed on me. I thought of my room upstairs, with its soft mattress and crisp sheets smelling faintly of lavender, and just hoped that Mum would ask for me to stay. Like any other child, I wanted to be tucked up, read stories and kissed goodnight and wake up to a smiling face.

Almost as soon as the video ended, Gran was back in the room. She sat down next to me, pulling me close, and said, 'Your mother's just told me how angry your dad was with you, but you know, Emily, you did nothing wrong.'

'They said I did,' I whispered.

'Well, that's because they were upset. But these are grown-ups' problems, not yours, and I'm sure that when your dad has had time to think a little, he will be sorry he shouted at you. Just give it a little time and you'll see everything will work out all right.'

A statement that I don't think either of us believed.

'Now,' she continued, before I could ask any questions, 'how would you like to stay here for a few days? Just so your parents can sort a few things out. Would you like that?'

For the first time that day, I felt a smile breaking across my face.

'Yes, please,' was my answer as I snuggled into the safe softness of her body. 'And Molly?' I asked, thinking of the little dog she had given me only a few months earlier.

'Of course you can have her here! After all, it was me who found her for you. I'll tell your mother to bring her over.'

Satisfied my little companion would be with me in the place where I felt loved and cared for, almost instantly I forgot about all the shouting and beamed at her.

Molly was, I thought, my best friend, one I hated being apart from. *She'll be here in the morning* was my last thought before I fell to sleep.

She wasn't.

Chapter 9

It would not take much to imagine just how upset I was the following morning when Mum returned with a bag of my clothes, but no little dog in sight.

'Where is she?' I asked pleadingly.

'Your dad's got her, said he would look after her while we're sorting a few things out.'

Now one thing you have to know about my mother is that she tells lies. Not that I knew that at the tender age of five, but before I was six, I had discovered it to be true.

Lies caused by spite, to get attention and lies to avoid trouble.

This lie, I found out later, was one of pure spite.

But then hearing Mum's excuse and remembering how much Dad had liked Molly – after all, it was he who took her out for walks – I believed her and tried to swallow my disappointment. Not that it stopped the tears prickling against my lids.

'Oh, don't start crying now, Emily! I've enough on my plate without having to cope with your sniffling. He'll tire of that dog soon enough and bring her back for me to look after.'

Before I could ask any more questions, she told Gran she had an appointment with the solicitors and could she lend her some money as she had to pay for the first interview straight away.

'Are you sure you want to rush this, Betty?' her mother asked, no doubt hoping for a few moments that maybe everything could be fixed or perhaps it was not as bad as she thought.

But Mum just shook her head and no more questions were asked, most probably because I was standing next to her.

The only thing I heard about that meeting was that he would have to pay – a sentence I heard repeated by my mother several times a day afterwards.

Chapter 10

Whatever Dad was due to give Mum, it could not have been enough, for after a couple of months she announced that she would have to find a job and while she was searching for one, I would have to stay most days at Gran's, something that suited me. Being with Mum with her continuous mood swings, either crying or cursing at me, had made the family home a place I was eager to escape from even more than usual.

Mum's family had suggested more than once that if she was finding it hard to make ends meet that she moved in with them. 'There's plenty of room,' Gran had said and she pointed out that she could look after me too. But it was an offer my mother declined. She had already made other plans, ones she did not wish to share with either her sisters or her mother – not that any of us knew what they were then. The child I had been was too young to put together the phone calls she overheard, but the adult me can.

As my aunts once said, Mum didn't like the word 'Miss' in front of her name. Or rather, she did not want to attend family get togethers without a man by her side. She might have played the sympathy card and revelled in all the attention, but pity was another thing. If her husband was living with another woman – who, let's face it, whatever anyone said, was a real stunner – then she herself did not intend to be single for long. Obviously, finding a man too quickly would mean she would not be getting all the attention and support she still needed so discretion was needed and a loose-lipped daughter might well be a problem so she readily arranged for me to spend even more time with her family. Though not too often, or they might have thought she was a neglectful mother – another name she didn't want bandied about. Not that out of earshot and sight, my mother had much time for me.

In fact, so much of that time is still clear in my mind. I can remember that miserable feeling of loneliness dogging me when it was just the two of us in our home: she made it crystal clear in so many ways that I was an irritating thorn in her side, her words not mine, and she didn't know what she had done to be burdened with me. But small children do not always take the hint to hide themselves away. Instead, as Mum complained, they got under her feet. I couldn't help myself trying to get her attention. Like all small children, I wanted to believe my mother loved me. Which no doubt is why I never blamed her for her bad temper.

Every time she snapped at me, I felt as if it was all my fault, that there was a reason she did not show me the affection my grandmother did. I knew she hated my fussiness with food, my refusal to walk on certain parts of the pavement and the way I twisted my hair and sucked my tongue for comfort. Those things I could not stop, but even so, I tried my best to be as good as possible. And all the time, I hoped I would be rewarded with a cuddle, even a smile – anything that would make me feel wanted.

Chapter 11

It certainly hadn't taken my mother long to decide that burdened with me or not, her life was not going to grind to a halt. On the mornings she told us she was job-hunting, I was deposited at my gran's. And the evenings when I was left with her family? 'I have to have a life,' I heard her saying. 'Going to meet some girlfriends.'

And what could my grandmother say to that?

Gran believed she was heartbroken by her husband's desertion and she needed her friends, didn't she, she told my aunts when they voiced their disapproval. I heard them, though, when my grandmother was out of earshot, saying they didn't think it was *girlfriends* their sister was interested in. What they didn't know about were the evenings when she left me in the house alone.

There was more than one time, when I watched unnoticed as she carefully applied make-up, that I knew my mother was going out and leaving me on my own. Catching me standing in the doorway, she would glare at me. 'Don't you open your big mouth and tell your grandmother I went out or you'll be in big trouble!' she spat out each time, before telling me to get back in bed where I belonged.

I can see the child I had once been now looking at her desolately, when in high heels and a clinging dress, she left the house in a waft of perfume while I took myself off to bed miserably. I just wanted her to do what my grandmother did: envelop me in her arms, kiss me on the cheek, say I was her special girl and then tuck me in.

Well, that was something that was never going to happen.

* * *

It took quite a while after my father had left before Mum came bursting through the door, cheeks pink with excitement, as she told her mother and sisters the good news. She had been offered a job in a restaurant, where she would be handling bookings, seating customers and generally making sure that everyone was being well looked after. Not only that, she had also found us a new place to live. Friends of hers, she explained, had bought their own council flat, but they couldn't sell it for five years and were happy to rent it out.

'They are off to Spain,' was the answer when Gran asked where they were going to live.

'And where is it?' My grandmother wanted to know and was clearly unhappy with the answer.

'Oh, but, Betty, that's the worst estate in the town!' she exclaimed.

'Well, not for long, not when people are buying their homes. Anyhow, it's all we can afford. Got to cut our cloth now, haven't we?' Mum told her snippily.

That was all I managed to hear of that exchange. I knew by the sudden silence it was a conversation that would be resumed only once I was out of earshot.

Chapter 12

I would not be telling the truth if I said my childhood was a happy one before *he* entered my life. After all, I had five years of living with two parents who gave me little time. Luckily for me, much of those early years was spent with my mother's family, who gave me the love I needed. But that didn't stop me from being aware that neither of my parents felt the same way as they did. If there were times I was unhappy, it was not something I talked about – I was used to being ignored. Maybe if I had understood just how bad my home life was, I might have told my grandmother. But not understanding, I said nothing.

How I wish I had, for soon after I turned five, Mum introduced me to the man who was to become my stepfather.

And Fear came into my life.

The moment I think of that day, a picture so vivid comes into my mind. I can almost see the pores in his skin, that shadow, so dark and smooth, it looked as though it was painted onto his jaw, his receding hair that made me think then of an inverted three and those eyes, pale grey and cold. Call it child's instinct, but I knew from the moment I saw him that I was never going to like him. In fact, what I felt was distrust mixed with just a tinge of fear and dread.

My mother, who never seemed to sense when I was unhappy, picked up on my aversion to the man she introduced as Carl straight away. Once she had me alone, she gripped the tops of my arms so tightly, the marks still showed when I went to bed. A stream of accusations spewed from her mouth – I was a jealous little girl, I did not wish her to be happy, I wanted her all to myself. Well, there was some truth in that, which is natural, though the last comment was a slight exaggeration. Just a little bit of her, an occasional smile, a pat on the shoulder, my name said with warmth, anything caring would have satisfied me.

If before the breakup she had seemed either indifferent or irked by my presence, since my father had left, there was anger on her face nearly every time she looked at me. If there was hurt and also loss inside her, to me she showed only the anger. I knew not only had Dad blamed me, but she did as well. After all, it was me, wasn't it, who had imparted that bullet of knowledge that had destroyed their marriage.

I did try to force my lips to smile at Carl the next time I saw him. Now adults might be able to plant phony smiles on their faces, but children have a knack of showing their real feelings very clearly. Right from the start, he saw that he was never going to turn me into his little admirer. Not being a man who was prepared to wait for what he wanted – in this case, a compliant child – he made it clear to my mother that I was creating a situation he could not tolerate.

This resulted in her tackling me again.

'You are to be polite,' she instructed me, 'and respectful.' He was to live with us. 'It was him that got us this flat and he's going to make it nice. He'll even do up your bedroom. He wants you to see him as your new father, so you'd better be grateful.' With that, she held my shoulders tightly and shook me, adding, 'Do you understand me, Emily? I'll not have you showing me up.'

I did, I understood all right: I would have to accept him and be respectful or I would be punished. And she would take his side, not mine – she wanted a man more than she wanted her daughter's happiness.

'So, are you going to be a good little girl, Emily?'

'Yes,' I whispered and got my first reward since my father had left – a quick hug.

* * *

Carl arrived the next morning. He was taking Mum out for the day, he told me. Not us, just her – I was going to Gran's. Seeing him in my mind still sends a shudder down my body for I cannot forget the expression on his face when, as he told me it was only the two of them going out, his eyes locked with mine in a deadly combination of obsessive ownership and contempt.

Chapter 13

My mother, wilful as she was about getting her own way, had enough sense not to move Carl in with us too soon. He might have been staying over on the nights I was forbidden to talk about, but their plan was that he would not take up full residency until he had gone through the hurdle of being introduced to the family. I heard her telling him that it was important to her that he met them and gained their approval first, which she had already arranged. All three of us would be going over to the aunts' houses in a week's time.

My heart sank at the thought of seeing him every day. It was bad enough that when he stayed over, he acted not only as though the place was his, but as if he had every right to tell me what to do. Worst of all, it was something Mum never pulled him up on.

'He's going to be your stepfather one day, Emily,' was all she said when I complained about him walking into my room and telling me off because I had my colouring books out.

'You should put them away neatly,' he told me, which was something, even in a bad temper, my mother never said.

Right from the beginning he had tested her reactions to him giving me orders. While he hoped there would be none,

I crossed my fingers to see if she would put me first. To begin with, it was just fairly good-humoured observations about something I was doing that he disagreed with. When he went a little further and criticised me more strongly for carefully arranging all the food on my plate, she still said nothing. Nor did she say anything at the next meal when he told me to stop playing with my food and eat it all up.

The next evening, I could feel him watching me as I pushed aside some meat that was too rare.

'She's far too fussy, Betty,' he remarked. 'I think you should just serve her the leftovers the next time she leaves something.'

And if I hoped she would tell him that she was used to that and it was no problem, I was to be disappointed. Yes, he was testing the water there all right. And how I hated that condescending monotonous tone to his voice each time he pointed out what he perceived to be my wrongdoings.

Not that Mum seemed to notice.

Each time I thought of what my life would be like when he was in the house full-time, I felt my stomach churn. It certainly would change, and not for the better, of that I was certain.

It was when I heard them talking about the flat that I realised why he treated our home as though it was his. My mother had told him that her family objected to the area we were living in – it was not considered a good area and they worried about the sort of children I would mix with.

'Well, they should be grateful a friend of mine was willing to give it to you at a reasonable rent, shouldn't they?' was his sneering response.

'That's not something I told them, was it?' she retorted.

'Don't worry, they'll think differently when I've fixed it up. It'll be like a little palace then, you'll see,' he told her in his reassuring voice – another one I already hated.

* * *

I never found out what it was he told my family about his background, and to me, it's still a mystery. The adult me believes he must have fallen out with his own family well before he came into our lives. Then there must have been some questions about where he lived, something I didn't know the answer to either. After all, it is usually the woman who moves into the man's home, not the other way around. I know one of his excuses was that as a single man he needed only a very small space, plus – and I winced when I heard him trotting this out – with all the upheaval in my life, moving again would be too disruptive for me.

That was something I had heard my mother repeat to my grandmother at a later date.

The day Mum arranged for Carl to visit her family fell on a Saturday when one of those big get togethers with a barbecue was planned.

'Everyone will be there,' she told him happily. 'That way, you will get to meet the whole family all at once and get it over with. After all, it's a bit much to trust Emily not to say anything, isn't it?'

That was her way of wrapping up a criticism inside a joke.

And what did Carl do to make certain he fitted in?

Made sure he learnt all about the interests of each of the adult members. And did not arrive either overloaded with gifts – 'too ostentatious' or too few – 'tight-fisted'.

Mum needn't have worried he would get that wrong – after all, he had wooed and won her in a suspiciously short time, hadn't he?

Out he went shopping the day before the gathering to return with two perfectly wrapped bunches of flowers for, as he said, 'his hostesses' and a carton full of beers for the men.

'Oh, I thought I'd better get your mother something too, Betty,' he added triumphantly, waving a large, but not too large, box of chocolates under her nose.

'Perfect, darling,' she murmured, throwing her shapely arms around his neck.

Ugh, gross! I thought.

*   *   *

The following day, Carl's welcome, when he presented his gifts, was almost as warm as Mum's had been. Evidently it was something Dad never thought to do as I heard my uncles mutter to each other later in the day.

Even worse as far as I was concerned, when Carl had shown his very recently acquired knowledge of football, my uncles turned to my mother, saying it looked as though she had found herself a decent bloke at last. He must have studied the sports columns for days before that family gathering for he was able to talk not just about the game and which team had played where, but also to name the players he admired as well.

Funny how they were exactly the same ones that the men in our family saw as their own heroes.

He even asked his hostess, Aunt Lizzy, if he could walk around her garden and then was able to name all the plants that grew in it.

Some research must have gone into that as well, I would say.

And me, he addressed more than once as 'sweetie'. Not that he ever called me by that name when we were out of the family's earshot.

Everyone lapped up his company, the women almost preening when he complimented them on their cooking. The men were happy to have another male in the family who shared the same interests as they did when he joined them around the flames as they cooked the meats.

There was one person though who did not warm to him – my gran.

I saw her watching him, her lips in a tight line. She was polite enough but if I sensed it at my age, I'm sure he must have done as well. He knew she had seen through him, seen the person he really was. It must have been then that he began to plan how he could rid both my mother and I of her influence.

A week later, he moved his cases into our flat.

'The furniture will arrive once the decorations are finished,' he told us.

Once those large feet of his were planted firmly under the table, he felt confident enough to start laying down the rules, rules that my mother seemed happy to agree with. Rules that over time were to make me his virtual prisoner. Not that there were locks on the windows or padlocks on the doors, but then there are other ways to turn a child into a captive.

I call them the bars of fear.

Chapter 14

Before *he* moved in with us, it was usually one of my cousins who fetched me from school and walked with me to my grandmother's. On the days she was seeing Carl, or 'working late', as Mum had told her mother, then I stayed happily overnight.

Gran's home was my refuge, it was where I felt safe the moment I walked in. Instead of being ignored or snapped at, I was greeted with a smile the moment I returned from school. Within a few minutes, I was sitting down in front of the TV to watch children's afternoon programmes. A slice of cake and a glass of lemonade were quickly placed on the small table beside me before I was left alone to watch my favourite cartoon characters. Giggling away at their antics, I could forget about everything, including *his* presence in my home.

All that began to change once he moved in.

He announced what his plans for my future were: 'I'm going to be your stepfather one day,' he told me, 'so I'm going to start acting as your father right now.'

'I have a dad,' I said and saw the darkening of his eyes.

'Well, he's not a very good one, is he? When did he last bother to see you?'

The day he left was the truthful answer. Mum had not told me when I would see him again, but my gran had tried her best to explain what was taking place between my parents. She had sat me down, her hand on my knee, and told me that things would change when everything was settled. Or rather, as I was a small child without any knowledge of the law, she said, 'When your mum and dad have sorted everything out, you will be spending some time with him. He really does want to see you.'

This was an adult's way of explaining to a small child that until the court made its custody ruling, Mum and Carl were refusing him any access to me. All I understood was that someday in the future I would spend some time with him and Lily. As I had no way of finding out how many times Dad rang Mum to ask to see me, I carried on believing that he did not visit because he did not love me.

A belief that my mother had cemented in, the day we moved to our new home. When everything was unloaded, I saw that the television was missing and asked where it was.

'Your dad came round last night and took it, said it was his. Anyhow, I asked him then if he wanted you to spend time with him and you know what the shite said? That he'd rather spend his time with the telly now he was getting it back. Nice, eh?'

The lump in my throat was too big to answer her.

So, when Carl made those comments and with Mum's words still lodged in my mind, I could hardly think of anything to say in Dad's defence.

It only took a couple more weeks for Carl to test my mother again. She had allowed him to lay down the rules and chastise me for any misdemeanors he could find.

I've labelled that Stage One.

Then came the start of Stage Two – seeing how she would react to him hitting me. To do that, he had to find an excuse. Or in his case, invent one, to justify his actions. For not only did he want to punish a child physically, he wanted Mum to admire him for it.

Education was the tool he chose as his weapon. It was important, he said, every time we sat down at the table together: 'Don't you agree, Betty?' And my mother, who I doubt had ever given it much thought, replied very firmly that of course it was.

First part of Stage Two achieved.

Carl was not interested in the fact that this was my first term at school and as I had only just started, I could hardly have learnt very much. Plus, there might just be a reason that five-year-olds are not given any homework – not that he agreed with that. It was something he voiced his opinion about very loudly when he questioned me about what I had learnt each day.

'As soon as children begin school, they should have some work set for them to do at home,' he stated, 'seeing as you don't seem to do much in the way of lessons there.'

'We learnt to tell the time today,' I ventured boldly.

Not that it had really seemed like a lesson to me, more of a game, with a big cardboard cutout of a clock with hands that our teacher moved before asking us to say what time it was.

'So, at least you can tell the time now. Let's see if you're telling the truth on that: what does 22 hours mean?'

But I had no idea and just looked at him blankly: surely there was not a 22 o'clock?

'So, you can't tell the time! Thought so,' he announced triumphantly when he saw my confusion. 'Anything else you can remember?'

'No.'

'Well then, you're obviously not learning enough there so I will have to help you, won't I? All right, before we get to that, you tell me what exactly you are learning at school that you think is important.'

Something told me not to tell him that there were two things I wanted to get right: the alphabet and spelling. I could already read – that I had learnt when my grandmother read to me. Every evening I stayed with her, out would come a book and she would bring alive the characters living inside it. The story I asked for most was of a little girl who fell down a very large hole before entering a world where animals spoke. As she read a chapter to me, I would peer at every word and then lock them in my head. Which meant it was the shape of words I recognised, not the letters. Something I kept quiet about. The teacher never asked the infant class if they could read, so I never said I could. And I was not about to tell him either.

'I like it when she reads to us,' was the only answer I could think of.

* * *

It was after that first inquisition that Carl announced another new rule.

During the week I was not to sleep over at my grand-mother's.

Both he and Mum would be back by five if not earlier and I was to be brought home from school once they rang and announced they were back.

'Your cousin Ben has already agreed to bring you. I'll give him some extra pocket money and he's fine with that. It gives your mother some time to get our supper ready if he brings you home.'

Or he did not want to face my grandmother every day, was my thought much later on when I got to understand how his mind worked a little more. Then, I just felt sick, knowing that he had already arranged this.

'We are a family now,' he told me, 'and that means we all sleep in the same house each night. Understood?'

I did, and my heart sank.

* * *

Once my stepfather had orchestrated that little loss of my liberty, he told my mother that he had no choice but to add some home schooling to my routine.

'She's clearly backward,' he said, 'and we both know that, even if your mother thinks she's bright. But unless we do something about it now, she will be dependent on us for the rest of our lives.'

Amazing what some adults will say in front of a child they think is slow in learning!

Those words worked all right. Mum just shrugged and told him she would be really grateful if he took over helping with my education as he was much cleverer than she was.

Chapter 15

My first lesson with him, I named 'Days of the Week' when I locked it away in my mind's filing cabinet. It was the first lesson he decided on when he found out that I was a bit wobbly when it came to naming every one of the seven days of the week. I knew Sunday was the day people went to church and Monday came after it, because then I went back to school after the weekend, but I was still unsure of the ones in-between. Up until he quizzed me, I had not thought it was important. My mistake, it seemed. With his finger wagging in front of my eyes, he told me in no uncertain terms it most certainly was.

'Now, let's see if you can get them right ... What's today?'

That one I knew, but the next one, when he asked what tomorrow was, I stumbled over.

'Try again, and get it right this time.'

Now before you ask how on earth I can remember the words he used each time I came home, when I had hardly turned five, it is because they were the same ones that left his mouth every time he stepped into his teacher role. Not that he would have lasted more than five minutes in today's schools. It would not have taken more than one day before a mob of angry parents came storming across the playground to get to him.

There he stood, towering over me, hands behind his back, looking as though he had just stepped out of a Dickens' book. Except I was not a boy and he was not holding a raised cane. Not that he needed one; his hands could inflict stinging blows on my legs as I found out when I forgot to answer Wednesday for the third time. And again, when I could not work out what the day after tomorrow was.

For five minutes, he shouted clues at me: 'Think of those stupid cartoons you watch. Now what days of the week are they on?'

'Schooldays,' I whispered.

His fist thumped the table.

'Are you being deliberately stupid, Emily? I mean, the names of the days! Now, what day comes after Monday?'

My mouth went dry and I could feel panic rising into the whole of my body and going right through me into my hands, which made them fidget and shake.

'Right, I think you need a little help in learning,' and his hand lashed out and slapped me hard across the legs.

Of course, I screamed, only to be told if I made that noise again then he would give me a good reason to make it.

'Now get those days right!'

Of course, I stuttered my replies, got them wrong and was slapped again and again until he gave up, leaving my five-year-old self trembling with shock.

'It's your family,' he shouted at my mother. 'Them spoiling and cosseting her has turned her into a retard!'

My mother finally lifted her head from the magazine she was flicking through.

'Oh, why do you always act so weird, Emily? Can't you get anything right?' she snapped. 'You listen to him!'

And I saw a gleam of triumph in his eyes, telling me if nothing else did that she was not going to support me. Carl knew it too. He had just gained her backing to punish me in whatever way he wanted. Spinning back to where I was standing, he grasped the back of my neck and squeezed hard.

'If you don't want to be a retard, you'll do as I say. *Retard*, Emily, that's what you'll be if you don't listen to me! Do you understand?'

All I understood was the pain I was feeling as his grip tightened. I didn't know what that word meant, but over the years as he repeated and repeated it, I soon learnt.

It's a word I never want to hear again.

Stage Two was completed.

Just remembering how he fired questions at me that he must have known I could not answer gives me a small shot of adrenaline. I can still hear that hectoring voice of his repeating them over and over as though the answers would suddenly appear in my mind. Not that he wanted them to. What would have been the fun in that? No, his enjoyment was in making me feel stupid and incapable of learning without his help.

But he was wrong, and as young as I was, there was something small and hard growing in my core, telling me that it was not me who was the stupid one. Even then it was that burgeoning certainty that helped me, though my knees shook nearly every time I was brought home from school and walked through that door.

Every waking hour I thought with such longing of how it had been before his arrival. All right, you will say, hardly perfect, but that hadn't stopped me before from being happy most of the time.

Chapter 16

I can't remember when it was that my mother insisted on my taking a pill every night. It might have been after the second or third time Carl had beaten me and she realised he found it too enjoyable to stop. I heard her telling everyone from my teachers and her family how clumsy I had become since I had grown a little – 'Always dropping things and bumping into doors and cupboards,' she said, more than once, followed by a light laugh, 'Well, that's kids like her for you, I guess.'

I saw a worried expression cross my grandmother's face when she heard those remarks: 'Well, I've not noticed anything,' was all she said.

Other people just seemed to see it as a running joke. 'If there's a hole, you can be sure she'll fall into it!' was another observation. This was told to everyone, from family and friends to teachers. Looking back, of course, she was beginning to cover up for him, for the bruises were showing.

I can't remember when Mum started buying arnica – maybe about a year later, when the beatings grew more severe. It became the one thing we never ran out of. There was the cream to put on bruises and the pills that were supposed to prevent them forming in the first place. I remember being given those pills daily. My mother told me they were vitamin pills to make me grow strong, but she didn't know I could read. Or that I was already adept at using a dictionary. I knew what they were before I was seven – they kept the bruising to a minimum.

A secret I kept to myself.

I liked the fact that I knew far more than he thought. My ambition was to ask him questions he could not answer. I knew that might take a few years but the thought brought me comfort.

Anything could make him punish me, coming home later than my mother and finding me watching my cartoons was one.

'Not going to happen in this house,' he said firmly before turning the TV off. 'Betty, what have I said? She's not to watch television, she has homework to do.'

Which I didn't, but there was no point in arguing with him.

Every day, I thought with such longing of how it had been before his arrival. That warm welcome at my grandmother's was the complete opposite of how he and Mum greeted me when I was brought back home: 'Oh, here you are,' was the best I got. It went without saying that there were no warm smiles and hugs, and that making me feel loved wasn't going to happen either.

Barely had I got through the front door than he, armed with questions, was waiting for me. He would wait a couple of minutes until my coat was off, even smile pleasantly, then tell me that Mum was cooking supper.

'Now, before we sit down, I want to know what you've learnt today,' he would add and the inquisition would begin.

We had been learning our times tables, we had done some simple arithmetic and practised the alphabet in the morning. In the afternoon, we listened to a story and then drew pictures so I only told him about the afternoon's lessons.

I was fooled that first time, but no longer. Not after he had mocked me about telling the time. I could have answered those questions if he had asked. I had gone to the teacher and she had explained what 22 hours meant: 'There are 24 hours in a day,' she told me, showing how the hands moved. So, now I knew.

That I had the answers to those questions gave me a little bubble of confidence. Not that I was going to tell him, any more than I let him know I could read. Now, I had two secrets, tucked away in my mind.

Not that they stopped my growing fear of him.

Every day, when the phone rang, telling me it was time for my cousin Ben to take me home, my stomach felt as though a lead brick had inhabited it.

Chapter 17

It's the week after Christmas and the house looks nothing like the pristine place my partner and I turned it into before his father arrived. Now, I do not turn my back on my children, but let's face it, no mother – and I don't care what anyone says – can watch them every second of the day.

Especially the one who at five considers herself old enough to tell me to go away!

So how long had Sonia been in her room, drawing a surprise picture for me? I asked myself, looking at one depicting brightly coloured falling leaves. Well, that's what I saw anyhow. Not for her the different height, stick-like figures showing how she sees her family, nor is there a picture of a cat nearly as big as me in it. Hers show, in bright colours, whatever it is we wish to see. In this case, falling leaves – they are also painted onto a wall that only the day before had shown a clean, blank surface.

Now, it has not been the first time we decided that washable paint might just work on the walls. I have tried to explain to Sonia that she mustn't draw on walls, except in her bedroom. Well, we had to do that, didn't we? We stiffen ourselves against her bewildered look. That in itself was a battle for us. Because hadn't I told her that her pictures were pretty and that I loved them? And then later, she had walked over to me and placed one in my hand: 'For me?' I asked and her reply was one of her beaming smiles that lit up her face and an enthusiastic number of nods. I had kissed her then and pinned the picture to the wall, where we could all see it.

Well then, if I like the pictures so much, why don't I want them everywhere?

Not that she says those words, I just know that is how she thinks.

Ever since she discovered crayons, she has drawn on walls, not colouring books. I understand why – she did not want them hidden away from us. She had even ripped off wallpaper to draw underneath it and the worst, when she was no more than three, somehow managed to pull a radiator off the wall. Thank goodness it was an electric one so no damage done to her or the wall – I think she thought it was too ugly to be on show. She had a point, I must admit, but still . . . Back on the wall it had to go.

It took a long time to explain why this was not one of her best ideas!

Of course, friends and relatives tell us she should be punished, that I'm far too soft with both of them. I try and explain that neither of my little girls understands what it is they have done wrong – they are wired up just a bit differently than us is how I see it. Naturally, they get punished if they've done wrong, but there's no physical punishment, insults or raised voices. And if I feel I was unfair, I always apologise. Just because I'm older doesn't mean I know better. Basically, I make sure that they grow up in an atmosphere which is the complete opposite of my own childhood.

But Patrick and I do speak very clearly when we need to lay down our house rules to the kids. Not that it always gets through. Seeing our disapproval is usually enough though. Mainly we just tell them not to do it again and fix it, for I never want my children to be afraid of adults who are over twice their size and never to crawl into bed, their whole bodies shaking with fear. So, I let Sonia paint and draw and if it gets on the clothes or furniture, I clean them.

No big deal. We create beautiful memories together instead of traumas.

So, in her bedroom I smile but as I do so, I feel my hand has reached for my hair. My fingers are twisting it so hard, it makes my eyes water, but I can't stop. Those drawings she's showing me with such delight have made another one of those dratted drawers spring open.

One labelled 'Punishment for Being a Liar'.

Well, I did say the Christmas period has its triggers that make my old fears easier to release. Oh, not the presents, the tree or the windows lightly dusted with December frost. No, it's not that, but certain words take me back to that part of my childhood and can set off my panic attacks.

So, let's just say this time it was the combination of the drawings and the season.

* * *

I see myself at six, just a short time after *he* moved in with us, living in such a dark, gloomy place that it gave me the creeps. 'All this flat needs,' *he* had said within a week or so of his boxes arriving in our hall, 'is a revamp.' That was his way of saying he was going to choose the colour scheme and fill every room with his dark furniture. Not one pretty thing was left – he had, in less than a week, exorcised any reminder of my mother's past life with her husband.

All the photographs had disappeared, little ornaments that once meant something to her departed with them and not one picture was left hanging on the walls. As for my bedroom, with its dark gold and burgundy striped wallpaper, I simply hated it. Even the lovingly made patchwork bedspread my grandmother had given me had been thrown out and replaced with a thick, dark plum coloured eiderdown that I felt smothered under.

Not that in the years I spent there, I ever felt it was my room. When I was little, no toys or colouring books were ever allowed to be left out anywhere. His head would suddenly appear around the doorway and if one small object was in what he thought was the wrong place, he took it away from me. When I was older and had real homework to complete, I tried to make it a place I was happy to work in, but the only concession he made to my changing my room around was to place a desk and a hard-backed chair under the window. Once finished, all paperwork had to be placed either in my satchel or in one of the drawers. And no, I couldn't hang a picture or pin up a poster. Even my pens had to be lined up neatly. As for books, there was a library, wasn't there? No more than two books were allowed in our house at any one time.

The flat was his domain and he controlled every part of it. And how had that come about? I simply couldn't understand how my once-bossy mother had become so subservient. It's as though once he came into our lives the badness within him seeped into her as well. I soon came to realise that she was not just putting up with his tyrannical behaviour, she was enjoying it.

'I'm doing it all for you and your mother,' he told us repeatedly when at weekends he rolled up his sleeves and armed with a variety of paintbrushes, commenced work. He decided we needed a nice place to live in, my mother would say proudly to both her family and me.

A pride she had never shown in anything Dad did when they were together.

Right from the start, I knew that when he said the flat had to look good enough for us, he meant good enough for *him*. God forbid he'd live somewhere that didn't look expensive or cost a lot!

Now I did say everywhere was dark, that is everywhere except the narrow hall that we almost had to squeeze through the front door to enter. For some reason he chose the palest wallpaper he could find, so pale it was nearly pure white, patterned with rows of faint blue dots. It hardly went with the rest of the house – not that I thought then that maybe it was there for a reason.

* * *

I was in my room feeling almost happy when I heard the front door open and knew he was in. *Just what lesson was he going to start on that evening?* The day before, it was sums and even though I had got everything right, he still yelled at me.

I knew it made him furious when I did well.

'*Idiot savant*,' he once called me. Then, gripping me by the arms, he leant forward, his face inches from mine. 'That means, Emily, that you are nothing but a clever idiot so don't think for a moment because you can add up, it means anything. Even an idiot can get one thing right!'

Good thing he hadn't found out I could read as well, I thought, when I heard the front door open and knew with a shiver that he was back.

What's going to happen tonight? I wondered, thinking for a moment that he was going to question me about my day at school. But something far worse occurred. The roar of rage that climbed up the stairs and into my ears told me to be wary of him.

'Emily, get yourself down here now!' he bellowed.

With shaking legs that barely held me upright, I left my room and went into the hall where he was standing, my mother at his side. I started to ask what was wrong, but before I had the chance, a firm grip on my shoulders turned me to face the wall.

'What do you see?' he asked, his finger pointing to a minute brown speck. 'You did that, didn't you?' he added, spinning me round to face him.

I hadn't a clue what he was talking about – the mark was hardly bigger than a pinhead.

Bending down so that his face was just inches from mine, he engaged in such intense eye contact that I wanted to close mine: 'You did it, didn't you?' And as I shook my head, I saw that red veil creep over his face and knew all hell was about to break loose.

I had seen his tempers before, received his stinging slaps each time he blamed me for something that had gone wrong – a dish left out in the kitchen, a coat not hung up – in fact, anything he considered a mess had to be my fault. This time, looking up into his hard, grey eyes, my stomach lurched: this was going to be far worse than anything else.

When he kept repeating what he thought the stain was, I knew I was in terrible trouble.

'It's your poo on there, isn't it? You little slut!' he yelled at me, running his finger along the wallpaper before holding it up to his nose. 'I can smell it, so don't deny it.'

With that, he spun me round again and pushed my face hard against the wall.

'You wiped your hands on it, didn't you? I know you did!'

No matter how many times I cried no, he still kept bouncing my head against the wall. It was only his hands holding my shoulders that prevented me from collapsing after he repeated that act a third and then a fourth time. I tried to glance at my mother – surely, she would come to my aid? Out of the corner of my eye, I saw an expression on her face I had never seen before. With a sinking feeling, I saw it was amusement at what he was doing. She was taking his side, but she must know I hadn't done it. Whether or not she did, I knew then there would be no help coming from her.

And then he did something that has lived with me all these years: he propped me up against the wall before removing his rings slowly, one by one, from those thick fingers of his.

'Take these, will you, Betty?'

And there was my mother holding out her hand for him to drop them in her palm. I saw her fingers curl over them before she moved away without saying a word. One of his hands shot out and seized me by the neck while the other slapped my face so stingingly hard, I stumbled back.

Left cheek first, then right.

Up until then his stinging blows had only landed on my legs. This was worse, much worse – he really wanted to hurt me. Through the pain I heard him repeating, 'Filthy little slut!' before catching hold of my hair and practically lifting me up in the air with it. Red-hot searing pain tore through my scalp and I screamed. A hand went over my mouth, muffling the sound as he dragged me along the hall towards the bedrooms.

'Right, now you're going to look at yourself while you keep repeating your lies,' he told me, releasing his hand from my mouth.

'Mum,' I screamed out, 'stop him, stop him!' but I only heard silence as her reply. I could not see her, but I knew she was there and then I heard a sound, the clip of heels as her footsteps moved away.

He dragged my sobbing younger self not into my bedroom, but into the one he shared with my mother. In there was a tall mirror propped against the wall. He stood me in front of it and although he kept his fingers twisted round a chunk of my hair, he released it slightly.

One move from me would bring back that searing pain.

'Now, who do you see in the mirror, Emily?'

'Me,' I managed to stutter out.

'No, you don't, you see a liar. Say it . . . say "I'm a liar".'

But I couldn't – I knew I hadn't put the stain there and I also knew it was not poo on the wall.

Another slap landed on my face.

'So, you don't think you're a liar? Well, look in that mirror again and tell me the truth. Now, what do you see?'

I saw a small child with tear-filled eyes and red welts in the shape of his hand on each of her pale cheeks. A child who was limp from fear and exhaustion while he, I knew, saw a victim – *his* victim.

'Well now, what would your grandmother think if she heard about this? Don't think she likes liars much either!'

At my young age, I did not have the vocabulary or the courage to say she would hate a bully more.

He shook me when it was clear I had no words left in me and told me to go to my room.

That day, I learnt it is not the truth that will set you free.

It took another ten years before I learnt what would.

I blinked, forcing that image of my younger self to recede. But not before another memory slunk in: my mother and him sitting together on the settee, laughing as they remembered the beating he gave me. 'Especially, that bit when it was wham, bam and then another slap!'

Now, that really cracked them up.

I could feel my heart racing at the memory, almost feel that old fear creeping back into me.

A small hand slipped in mine. Blue eyes in a smiling face with the flawless skin, fine and delicate as mine had been when he marked it, looked up at me.

Not the time for a panic attack, I told myself. *Sonia is waiting.*

Taking a deep breath, I straightened my shoulders and pulled myself back to the present day. Looking back at my daughter, with that expectant expression as she waited for me to praise her artwork, I smiled down at her.

'It's lovely, darling,' I said.

For didn't I want her to have only happy memories to look back on when she left childhood?

Chapter 18

Carl had won, there was no doubt about that. I would say every move he made from the first day he met us had been well thought out. From even before he tested my mother's reactions to him ticking me off to when he raised his game to physically punish me. I've heard of children being groomed, but it's only since the drawers started flying open and I had another look at those early years that I realised that adults can be too. But then perhaps I should have taken more notice of some of the cases that have made headline news.

You know the ones – seemingly ordinary women meet men whose hobby is inflicting suffering on those who are smaller and defenceless. And what happens? Evil seeps into them until they too wear the label marked 'monster'. I have studied Psychology at college, but never found the answers to explain just how these people are able to transfer their darkness into another. How Carl did it, I will never know – not even with my first-hand knowledge of seeing it unfold right under my nose.

It had certainly not taken him long to progress from telling me what to do to hitting me so badly, I was just about traumatised. If I was aware of Mum's barely concealed amusement when she watched those actions, then he must have been as well. And what had that told him? Not just one thing, but two.

He had managed to bring out something in her which made them almost kindred spirits. Not that I understand how he was so sure he could manage to achieve that when he first met not just Mum, but me as well. In less than a year of him moving in, he had completed the first two stages of his plan and was confident that he was now ready to take the next step: progressing from physical to what anyone else but my mother would have called sexual abuse. Or, as I would put it, Stage Three could then commence.

I feel now that he had known exactly what he wanted that very first day he had met me – a small plaything he could totally control and abuse, even though he was almost certainly aware that he could not go too far, too early on. The type of abuse he had in mind would have to start off quite subtly to begin with – little games that I would at first believe were just that. After all, this was not the dark ages of a few decades earlier, where abuse was never talked about, or if it ever came to light, then it was the child who became the pariah in society. This was the nineties, where social workers, police and teachers were beginning to be trained to deal with any suspicions of abuse, including physical as well as sexual. Goodness, if only I'd been able to speak out, they would have had a field day all right! But I didn't, for I had no way of knowing that a child giving a detailed description of her mother's lover touching her inappropriately would be listened to. Not only listened to, but action of some kind would be taken swiftly. Childline – the confidential service where children can talk about anything – was out there and now the public was becoming aware that all too often it was a trusted family member who used his position to groom or threaten youngsters into accepting years of abuse.

Not that I ever heard about that organisation until I was a lot older. I'm certain both Carl and my mother were fully aware of it and made sure that I never saw their phone number when it flashed up on the TV screen.

I doubt that Carl was overly concerned about me talking though. By then I think he was utterly convinced that I had become far too afraid of him to risk it – and he was right. In fact, I was more than just frightened, my new shadow was Fear. It had let me know it would be my constant companion and promised never to leave me while I lived under my stepfather's roof.

I've heard Fear described in many different ways, from lurching stomachs, shaking, sweats to fast-beating hearts. But that's panic, not the deep-rooted fear I'm talking about. How I would describe it is as a white empty space forming in the mind where that little demon takes up residence gleefully. Once safely ensconced, it will stop all independent thinking and all reasoning ability. When it chooses a battered woman's brain, she seldom leaves her fist-wielding partner for Fear mutters incessantly that she was to blame for him losing his temper. And wasn't he sorry afterwards, didn't he tell her he loves her more than anyone else would? So, believing no one else will ever feel the way he does for her, she pulls on her long-sleeved tops to hide the bruises and tells everyone about that stupid door that blackened her eye. There is even a novel about it – Roddy Doyle's acclaimed work, *The Woman Who Walked Into Doors.*

Now, I do know from both the newspapers and the news that there are some who find the courage to make their escape – the ones who recognise a monster when they see one. Some find a refuge that will protect them, others run as far away as possible and then there are a few who snap and pick up a knife, a hammer or whatever comes to hand, to batter or stab their partner to death.

Even our country's prisons are safer than the one they have been living in.

But you need to realise that I'm talking about an adult's brain. When Fear enters a child's brain, it's far easier for it to take complete control. Once inside their head, its spider-like tentacles reach out to take over their thoughts, speech, even their limbs. If that's not enough, it trespasses into their dreams, turning them into nightmares.

It's a peculiar thing that children find one of the worst threats made to them is not being beaten, but being taken away and put in a home where both the windows and doors are locked. They are told when that happens they will never, ever see their family again. Like the child I was, they are even more afraid of losing the very people who are cruel to them – they just want the bad things to stop. Which means the fear of being ripped away from every-thing they know is strong enough to silence them. Like me, they have been told not to talk – so they don't.

That is one of the problems that social workers have to deal with. Like my dad, and my grandmother, they might suspect something is wrong, but little can be done when they are faced with a child who denies it. And in my case, as I'm sure it has been for all the silent others, the abuse gradually became almost a daily ritual.

Another trick that Carl put in play was aimed at confusing his victim. Maybe if I'd been allowed to just simmer with hate during my childhood, that would have been easier. But no, he turned me into someone who wanted to gain his approval. That way, he was able to control me even more. He really perfected that part of his plan to a tee. Little deeds of kindness followed by praise to make me feel almost special. Trouble is, when that happens so seldomly, the victim begins to feel grateful for just a few crumbs of attentiveness – sad, but true.

He would be all smiles and friendliness, sometimes for a day, sometimes even longer. Then just for that short time I would begin to feel safe. He would tell me he loved me, that he saw me as his daughter and that the lessons were only there to help me, that he wanted what was best for me. Sometimes he would even buy me little gifts (some hair ribbons, a pencil case once and the odd bag of sweets), read to me and even allow me to watch TV with him and Mum once or twice.

Those times made me almost forget, though not quite, about the little demon living inside my head. And once he was sure that I'd slipped under his spell, with warm smiles and a look of interest on his face, he began to take an interest in a hobby of mine – my painting.

Apart from being an avid bookworm, like my daughter, I have enjoyed both painting and drawing ever since I was old enough to hold a crayon or a paintbrush in my hand. Today, it's something Sonia and I often do together. It's always more fun for a child, isn't it, when another person admires what they're doing? It gives me such pleasure when I see her eyes sparkling with happiness each time I praise her on one of those occasions when I have managed to persuade her to paint on paper in the hope that she will continue to stick to that.

Not that this was what Carl encouraged me to do. *Oh no, he had a completely different idea! To paint on skin – his.* An idea that must have formed in his head when he saw me drawing little pink stars on my arms. If I was unable to resist using the background of my pale skin as a canvas then I could also use his too, couldn't I, he told me magnanimously. Especially as more than once he had watched me extend my drawings to my legs as well.

This *was* something my mother objected to, even though it was easy to wash off. To my surprise, for once Carl took my side and said it was OK with him: 'It looks pretty,' he said laughingly.

I was certainly fooled by that burst of good humour as I was when he came home with an assortment of paints and some more brushes.

'Maybe she can train to be a tattooist,' he told Mum. 'You only have to have a good eye for that and then plenty of money comes in!'

She didn't make any comment.

I was so busy admiring all the paints he had put in front of me that his words went straight over my head.

'Do you know what that means?' he asked me and I shook my head. 'It's drawing beautiful pictures on people's skin. Some people are covered everywhere with them – their arms, their necks, even their backs. Now, let's see how well you can paint on me as well as yourself,' he suggested, rolling up his sleeve. 'After all, it will save on paper, won't it?'

At this I heard an underlying amusement in his voice which made me feel uncomfortable without understanding why. I might not have come to like him, or even trust him, but it still made me feel good when he admired what I was doing. To begin with, he made me paint pictures on his arms, which was almost fun. Though I did not like touching the dark hair that grew on them. Not that he was satisfied with that for long.

'Come,' he said, once I had drawn the same stars on his wrist that I had painted on mine. 'I think we can do a little more, don't you? Let's see what you can draw on the top of my arm.'

Rolling his sleeve up a little further, he pulled a towel under it.

'There you go, it's a blank canvas.'

Not blank enough, though.

I remember looking at it with something like revulsion – my skin was clear and light while with his sleeves rolled up, all I could see was that thick, dark hair. I wanted to pull away but his eyes bored into mine, holding me there.

'Come on, Emily, I'm waiting for you . . .'

Obediently, I dipped my brush in one of those small pots and painted on a dark blue circle.

That was a start of something I did not understand, not then.

Now, I do.

When he appeared bored with circles and flowers on his arms, he suggested I try on his legs.

Legs were longer, weren't they?

To begin with, it was just the rolling up of his trousers; his eyes would flick between my mother and me. And when she appeared only amused, the trousers were rolled higher . . . until the day he decided to take them off.

Still, she said nothing.

A rug was placed on the floor and I, fighting back something I had not a name for, did as he asked and painted away on his legs.

'Higher,' he told me.

Bracing myself, I did as he said. When I had covered his legs and then his back with paint, I sat back, exhausted at doing something that so revolted me. That was when he announced, 'Shower for us! Got to get this paint off, haven't we?'

It slowly dawned on me that he meant both of us together.

I looked up at Mum, hoping she would not agree to such a thing.

'Your dad will take you,' was all she said.

I wanted to say something, ask her to take me. Young as I was, I was fussy about who helped me shower – I didn't want him to see me undressed either.

'Oh, just run along, will you?' she said impatiently.

Powerless to do anything else, I followed him out of the room.

That first time he got in with me, rubbed soap on my body and then asked me to do the same to him. I hated having the water pouring down on me. *Didn't they realise it stung?* Not only that, the steam was making it hard to see and I was scared the water would get in my eyes. That was something that really scared me, so I closed my eyes and kept ducking my head.

Not that I wanted to look at his body so close to mine. There was that thing sticking out that I didn't want to touch. I knew what it was – I had too many little male cousins not to know it was how they peed. But his was much larger than theirs.

That first time we were both in the shower, he didn't touch me in those places I thought of as private, he just lifted me out, wrapped a towel around my body and rubbed me dry.

'Pop off to your room and get your pyjamas on,' he told me. 'I'll make you a cup of hot chocolate.'

That's what I mean – he was capable of those little acts of kindness.

Of course, I know the word for what he was doing now. *It's called grooming.*

I would like to say it stopped there.

It didn't.

Chapter 19

I had no idea of the repercussions that a small act of mine would cause.

It happened one day when I was visiting my grandmother after school. My parents actually rang and told her they were delayed so I could stay a little longer. They had already asked Ben, my mother told Gran, and my cousin was OK about making the journey a little later.

I heard my grandmother offering for me to stay the night but it was clear from her response of 'Oh, all right then,' that Carl was sticking to the rule of no sleepovers during the week. Not that it happened very often on weekends either – another reason for me to resent him and all those rules of his.

I can't remember why I was standing in the kitchen just under a shelf – I have only the memory of one of my uncles raising his arm to lift something down from it. I didn't see my good-natured uncle getting something down for Gran, what I saw instead was a large hand wearing a thick gold signet ring on his little finger, raising above my head. Fear suddenly stirred from its slumbers and screamed out at me, *It's going to come down and hit you on your head and send you crashing to the floor again!* I raised my arms instinctively to ward it off and a whimper left my mouth as I cowered against the wall.

'Whatever is the matter, Emily?' my gran asked, moving swiftly towards me. 'Come here,' she added softly and her arms enveloped me and held me tight as I burst into tears.

I could hear my uncle talking and Aunt Lizzy asking what he'd done to frighten me so, but everyone in the room knew that it wasn't him who had caused me to be so upset. As the word 'bruises' was mentioned, I heard a few shocked gasps.

'I said our Emily had changed since Betty met that man,' my uncle stated.

Gran shot him a look, one that told them all that they must choose their words carefully as I could hear them.

'Come on, darling, there's nothing to be frightened of here,' my grandmother whispered in my ear.

Using all my willpower, I managed to stifle my sobs.

'Now, tell me what upset you so,' she continued once she saw I was calmer.

But Fear refused to be quiet; instead, it told me to say I didn't know and those were the words that I repeated to Gran.

'You know you can tell us anything? You won't get into any trouble here. You know that, don't you? So, is there anything you want to tell us, Emily?' she asked.

'No,' I whispered.

Good old Fear – it certainly knew how to shut a child up all right.

My grandmother said little more about what had frightened me. A few minutes later, the phone rang, making me shake. I knew without asking that it was them summoning me back home.

I wanted so badly to stay where I was, wanted to tell Gran what had frightened me so much, beg them not to send me back, but Fear quickly blocked my words as it murmured, *Think of the punishment you could get if you talk.*

'Don't say anything, will you?' I whispered to Gran.

'No, of course not, darling. It was just a misunderstanding, wasn't it?' she said.

Looking up at her, I saw a mixture of concern and anger in her eyes before she quickly changed the subject: 'This is the first weekend that you'll be staying with your dad, isn't it?'

It was something I was nervous about. I hadn't seen him since he'd walked out just over two years ago and hadn't I heard repeatedly that was because he didn't love me as much as Carl did? It was only because the courts had told him that he had to take some responsibility that he had agreed to have me to stay.

At that age I was unaware that this was another of Mum's lies. How I wish I had known that in fact Dad had to fight both Carl and my mother in court to obtain shared custody. And who had spoken up for him – Gran. She had said whatever the differences between her daughter and her former partner, she only ever witnessed him being a good father.

No doubt another reason Carl was wondering how he could separate Mum from her family.

* * *

The one bright spot on the horizon about the arranged visit was that I was going to see Molly again. She wouldn't be a puppy now for she must have grown over the months since Mum had told me my father had her – I just hoped she hadn't forgotten me.

Not that, for some reason, I mentioned her to Gran when she said, 'I expect you're looking forward to seeing him, aren't you?' A question I managed to say yes to, though it was not completely true. My answer, I noticed, placed an expression of something like relief on her face.

When she helped me on with my coat, she just said, 'You know we're always here for you, don't you? Any problems, you come to me.'

'Yes,' I said and received another hug before she handed me over to Ben to escort me home.

I had heard Aunt Lizzy saying maybe one of them should take me this time but Gran shot them a warning look and said, 'Later, we'll talk about that later.'

Ben must have heard what had happened – I should think the whole family knew about it by the time I left. I expect he had been asked to try and persuade me to confide in him. For once he didn't call me 'Sprat' or come out with any of his usual gentle teasing. Instead, he wrapped his hand round mine.

'Look, Emily,' he told me gently, 'is there anything you want to tell me? We're friends, aren't we? And friends can tell each other everything.'

Don't even think about it! screeched Fear. *Don't trust him, he'll just repeat it all to his parents.*

So, I ducked my head, unable to bring myself to look at him when I said, 'I'm all right.' I knew he sensed that I was holding something back. He clearly knew I was still upset and squeezed my hand gently, but that didn't stop me noticing that the expression on his face was the same as I had seen on Gran's.

Once home, it was my mother who opened the door to us.

'Oh, thanks for bringing her back. Come on in, won't you, Ben?' she said brightly.

'Can't,' he mumbled. 'Got homework to do.'

Placing a hand on my shoulder, he said, 'Night, Sprat,' then turned and walked away, leaving a void in the space he had occupied.

*   *   *

If I had thought my gran would simply forget what had happened, I was wrong. That evening, she rang Dad and offloaded her concerns down the line. Now, of course I don't know exactly what was said, but I can imagine she was blunt enough – Gran was never a woman to mince her words. Certainly, the family believed Carl was guilty of hitting me.

I know she told my father about that evening and no doubt voiced some of her suspicions as well. The Court ruling now allowed him access every other weekend. Luckily, he was due to pick me up from school that Friday. I expect he told her that he would try to get to the bottom of my being so upset then.

Not that those alternative weekends always happened, as neither Lily nor my parents were enthusiastic about those stays.

Both sides came up with various excuses ranging from a birthday party in my mother's family to Lily having a dose of flu and then the final excuse of Lily's that sent Mum into an apoplectic rage – morning sickness, Lily was pregnant.

Still, neither side had been able to come up with a good enough excuse for that first weekend. Mum, true to form, made it clear that she was surprised at my father wanting to see me – 'I suppose it's to get back at me,' she said with a grimace when she told me about the arrangement.

Trust Mum to think that it was all about her!

'Anyhow, good luck to you, sleeping there with that slut! And having to be nice to the man who walked out on both of us. But you go, if you want to.'

'Betty, she doesn't have a choice, does she? He has a legal right to see her,' said Carl as he walked into the kitchen. 'We just want you to remember we're your family, Emily, the ones who love you. Isn't that right, Betty?'

'Of course it is,' she agreed, giving me a quick hug.

'So, don't forget that, will you, Emily? We're going to miss you,' he persisted.

'We certainly will,' Mum said breezily.

All I can say is that children have very short memories, or perhaps they can easily be made to believe what they want to. Because on hearing those words, I started to feel a warm glow inside me.

* * *

I took my overnight bag to school. Clearly, Mum didn't wish to see my dad's face at the door. When I walked through the gates later that day, there he was waiting for me.

'Hello, Emily,' were the first words he spoke.

If I was hoping for a hug or an 'Oh, how I've missed you!' I was due for a disappointment. But then my father wasn't someone who showed much emotion.

It's a shame that when I met him that day, I had no knowledge of how hard he had fought to get joint custody. If I had, I might have felt more secure, more loved by him. Then maybe I would have talked to him.

Sadly, I didn't.

He picked up my overnight bag and walked with it to the car.

'I thought we could go to a coffee shop, spend a little time together,' he told me. 'You still like ice cream?'

Well, what child can resist that offer? Certainly, not me – not at that age, anyway. Though the fact he clearly wanted a chat with me was surprising. That was not something he had requested very often, or to be honest, at all. There was something about me that seemed to unnerve him. As I grew older, I realised that he was not the only one I had that effect on.

Once we were settled in the coffee shop and half of the three scoops of ice cream were already sliding down towards my stomach, he leant across the table and asked if I was happy at home.

'What do you mean?' I said, playing for time.

'Is your mother's man good to you?'

And there was my escape route. *Tell him*, said a voice inside my head, *tell him about the beatings, tell him about him wanting you to touch his body and tell him about the showers.*

And then what will he do? asked Fear and my mind went blank.

It was Fear that made my stomach clench and removed my voice from my throat.

'Come on, you can tell me, I'm your dad,' he persisted. 'Is there anything wrong at home?'

And what would you do if I told you? was the next question that flew into my head.

Ring Mum to confront her and she would deny everything. Then she would tell Carl and he would just about kill me.

Too young and too frightened to recognise the Get Out of Jail card lying in front of me, instead I allowed Fear to cement in another bar of the prison that Carl was busy creating.

'No, everything's all right,' I said.

'Really?'

He looked at me hard as he asked and I dropped my gaze to the bowl.

'Yes, really,' I said, spooning another lot of ice cream into my mouth.

Change the subject, Fear told me. *Ask him about Molly. Ask how she is because you'll be seeing her soon.*

So, I did, only to see a blank look appear on his face.

'What did your mother tell you?'

I saw a flash of temper flicker in his eyes as he asked.

'That you took her and the TV,' I managed to say, for I could feel a coil of dread unravelling inside me.

He was quiet for a moment and I think I knew already what he was going to say.

'Look, Emily, your mother lied about that. OK, I took the television, it was a rental and it was in my name, but not your dog.'

'Then, where is she?'

I guess now that he had no idea where she was. Most probably, my mother had dumped her at a refuge, but Dad wanted to give me some words that would console me a little.

'Look, she told me she couldn't manage and that she had found her a really good home.'

'Then I could visit her, couldn't I?' I asked, tears threatening.

He sighed and picking his words carefully, said, 'I don't know where they live, the family who have her.' He then tried to reassure me again that she was being well looked after.

Deep down, hadn't I known ever since my mum turned up without my puppy that Dad hadn't got her? She never liked the bother of having her in the house – not that she could tell my gran that. Her opportunity came when Dad left: she could blame him and appease her mother. But by then, I guess Gran already knew – nothing much escaped her gaze.

Dad didn't ask me any more questions about Carl, just tried to make conversation about school, then we went back to where he lived.

I can't say Lily's welcome was a warm one – in fact, she seemed pretty pissed off at having me to stay. Paul, on the other hand, was happy enough.

Once we were in his room playing, I asked him if what my dad had said was true.

'He never brought Molly here,' he told me. 'But I heard him on the phone tell your mother she was a bitch, giving your puppy away.'

So there was my answer.

Did I tackle her? No, knowing what she had done was another secret I kept tucked away. She must have wondered if he had told me the truth, but I was not going to give her the satisfaction of having to justify it.

Dad did not bring it up again. When he took me home on the Sunday morning, I glanced at him, wondering if he was going to walk me to the door. Instead, he handed me my case, told me he would see me soon and then got back in his car.

'See you soon,' he said with such a warm smile that I wished I had told him that I had missed him.

Dad might not have wanted to face my mother or Carl, but that didn't stop him ringing her.

How do I know?

She was foolish enough to tell me.

She asked me what I had told him about Carl and looked relieved when I just said, 'Only that he helps with my lessons.' That's when I knew that if he wasn't scared of my talking, she certainly was.

The short-term benefit for me now seeing my dad was that the beatings stopped for a while. In fact, it seemed Mum and Carl were going out of their way to be pleasant. He even brought home a present for me – a bicycle.

I should have known when he used the word 'teach' as opposed to 'show' that learning to ride my new bicycle was not going to be the treat Carl had made it out to be. However, I was still too thrilled at having that present to pay any thought to how I was going to learn to ride it. Lost in my daydream of joining my cousins on their bike rides, I had not taken in the word which normally broke me out in a cold sweat.

I had watched two of my younger cousins learning how to master that two-wheeled machine. One of them stood behind the other holding the saddle as they learnt to balance. Then wobbling all over the place, they had managed a few yards before starting all over again. By the end of the day, whooping away with glee, they were pedalling on their own – that's what I hoped was going to happen to me. Though

I did wonder why he wouldn't let me practise nearer our home. I knew he had said he wanted to go where there was no traffic, but we could have gone over to my aunt's house and used their driveway – that would have been a safe place to learn. But no, he wanted to make it a morning out in the fresh air and told my mother and I to wrap up warm.

Mind you, I should have guessed that Carl was not going to make learning to ride a bike easy – that was not his style. It was just that he had been so nice to me for several days that my defences were lowered so I didn't pay much thought to how he was going to do it when I climbed excitedly into the back of the car. But then, I had not yet worked out all of his controlling methods. One was to be so angry with me for several days that I quaked with fright, making me feel then that there was nothing I could do right and I must be as stupid as he kept telling me I was. Then, just when I was feeling as low as it was possible to feel, he would suddenly change and be affable and praise me. And what was my reaction? I began to crave those times when he smiled at me and told me I was special. So, every time he lost his temper, I blamed myself, even when I felt deep down that I had done nothing wrong.

It took me a long time, but eventually, I worked out exactly what his game was: be nice, praise Emily and then be angry and let her spend a couple of days doing every-thing she can to win back that nice, smiling person he had the art of showing her. I know now, looking back on that day in the woods, what his aim was – to make me seem ungrateful.

A failing that he would be able to berate me for endlessly.

Unaware of any of that then, I smiled back at him when he asked, still in his warm, friendly voice, whether we were both comfortable. Receiving a yes from each of us, he responded cheerfully, 'Right, off to the country then!' as he started the engine and pulled away.

My excitement quickly drained away when he drove into a densely wooded area. Glancing around, I saw, under the thick canopy of leafy branches, what lay around me – thick bushes, broken stone walls and steep paths covered with fallen twigs and branches.

'Now, here's a good place to start,' he told me, as he took my bicycle out of the boot. 'I'm going to choose a path for you that's easy and we'll see how you get on, all right?'

What could I say? Not that I thought for one moment it was going to be all right. Up until I saw those rocky, twisting paths, his good humour had tricked me into believing that this was going to be a fun day out.

Just try and stop yourself from falling off, muttered Fear, *you know he'll like it if you do.*

* * *

Carl made it clear that I was to manage on my own right from the start. No holding the saddle until I felt ready to go it alone. Instead, with me pushing the bike behind him, he walked up to the top of a steep slope. Not that it was too high, thank goodness, or I might not be telling this story.

'Now, up you get,' he told me.

I tried to sit on the saddle and put my feet on the pedals, but I wasn't ready – I had no sense of balance. Hastily, I placed one foot on the ground to prevent myself falling.

'Try again, Emily,' he said and this time he held the saddle while I clambered back on.

If I had thought he was going to continue to do that while I pedalled, I was wrong.

'Right,' he told me and then without warning, gave it a firm push and launched me down the hill. Of course, I was going too fast. Panicking, I clutched the brake hard and sailed into the air, the cycle falling down beside me.

My elbow hurt, my knee was bleeding, but did either of them come rushing down to see if I was all right? *No!* Instead, Carl just shouted from the top of that slope for me to push the bicycle back up. I forced myself to get up and swallowed my tears – they were not going to get me anywhere.

'Now,' he said, 'the thing is to get straight back on, show who's in control. Don't start grizzling, you'll thank me for it later.'

I didn't, not ever, because by the end of that day, I had begun to understand just what he was doing.

My next attempt at controlling the bike ended up the same way. The third attempt had me landing in a thorny bush and on the fourth, I ended up bouncing off a crumbling stone wall.

It might have been the end of that so-called fun day out, but it was not the end of me. That little kernel, growing inside my core, the one that had told me that I was not the stupid one, managed to resurface.

Conquer that bike, Emily, or he will have won again, it told me.

For once Fear knew its place and kept silent.

I bit my lip – I wasn't going to cry, nor limp nor complain. Without saying a word, I moved the bike away from where he could push me in the direction of another bush, tree or wall.

Putting one foot on the ground to steady myself, I got on it again.

Concentrate, I told myself.

It took more than one attempt to manage to stay on it, but by the end of that day, I was able to control the bike. I cycled down that first path he had chosen for me and then pushed it up to the top triumphantly.

Sore I might have been, but that didn't stop me feeling some pride in myself.

I had stopped him winning.

He managed to praise me and of course, took all the credit for teaching me his way. But this time I wasn't fooled – I saw the gleam in his eyes that told me he was heading towards one of his dark moods. It would not take long for him to look for any excuse to criticise me.

At least on that day, I felt it was worth it.

My memories of his bike-riding lessons are of being hurt. It was, I knew, down to me that I had refused to be traumatised. Carl's and my mother's memories though seemed completely different. As I grew older, I heard them recount what they felt were fond memories of different lessons he had given me. There were lots of laughs and gestures from them.

'Well, thanks to me,' he would say with a smirk each time, 'you know the days of the week and you can ride a bike. I hope you're grateful.'

My response was a forced smile – I had learnt at a young age to hide my true feelings.

Chapter 20

For several days after that bike incident, I could feel Carl's barely suppressed temper simmering away – although he should have been more cheerful, as I was clearly too scared to talk. There had been more than one opportunity that he knew of for me to have talked, hadn't there? Both at my grandmother's and over the weekend I had spent with my father.

He really must have been feeling so smug at the success of the three stages he had engineered. Now he was living with a woman who let him do as he wished with her daughter and a child who had shown she was completely under his control.

The result of his complacency was that those crazy, despotic rules of his increased on a daily basis, from leaving my shoes at the door to writing down everything I had done at school. He searched those notes hopefully for spelling mistakes and patrolled my room to ensure I had not left one thing out in my bedroom. Whatever rules he had made for my mother, I was not party to – though I'm sure there were some.

I could feel his hold over us growing stronger and stronger. Once he was confident that Mum had no objection to him hitting me, or in other words, her silence showed her acceptance of it, he used any excuse to raise his hand to me. Not only that, but even worse was seeing how much pleasure he took in taunting me with what was to come. He had his own way of preparing for the beating he was going to administer, preparations that became increasingly frightening.

First, he would accuse me of some wrongdoing, however minor, such as leaving a book out in my bedroom. It made no difference – he had already decided what he wanted to do. Once he had vented enough anger in my direction, he would tell me to fetch a saucer from the kitchen, then very slowly take off his rings, one at a time, before dropping them in the saucer that my shaking hands were holding.

Every ping made by metal landing on the china made me shiver and my back muscles twitch at the thought of how much I was going to be hurt. I knew why he took those rings off – they would have torn my delicate skin had he not. Recognisable marks left by them might just raise questions at the school and certainly would if Gran spotted them. This explained why, most of the time, he was careful not to leave marks in the wrong places. Bruises on legs could be dismissed by saying I had knocked against some furniture but a swollen cheek with red fingermarks on it or a black eye, now that would be a different matter.

Unluckily for me, the backs of my legs – the area he concentrated on most of the time – felt just as much pain as any other part of the body. There were only a few occasions where, when his loss of temper was genuine, then not marking me in the wrong place went out of his head. Then blows rained down on whichever part of my body was the nearest to his fists.

It was Mum who shouted at him when she saw he was out of control. The first time I heard her raised voice, I had believed that she was trying to stop him, that she was actually standing up for me. Then I wasn't listening to the words leaving her mouth. Once I was a little older, I heard quite clearly what they were – 'Carl, your rings' – and then I knew who her concern was for.

By then I had discovered that I was not the only one using arnica. I saw how the tube the cream was in had less in it than when I had used it previously. I'm sure, if I could have counted the tablets, I would have found some of those missing too. She really didn't have a clue how much I had worked out about what went on in our home. I'd heard his raised hectoring voice through my bedroom walls. There were nights when I was woken to my mother's cries and his angry shouting. Sometimes I would curl up as tight as possible under the blankets, trying to muffle those sounds by placing my fingers in my ears. Other times, I would creep along the corridor and stand outside their bedroom. I recognised the sound of flesh hitting flesh all right. Not that Mum ever said anything, whatever bruises she had were well covered.

Did she really believe that all the rooms in the flat were soundproof? And didn't she think I might notice sometimes when a sleeve rode up to reveal a circle of bruises on her arms, or how, on more than one morning, she walked stiffly as though every step hurt. I noticed all of that as well as how pale she often looked and how she frequently winced with pain.

As a child, I could not understand why my mum accepted his tyranny. She was still the mother, who only a short while ago had nagged and nagged at my dad – a man who never laid a hand on either of us. He might have clenched his fist and thumped the wall in frustration when she refused to stop nagging, but that was as far as it went. His escape was not violence – it was to refuse to answer her, or to leave the house muttering he was leaving to meet up with friends.

There were times when Carl's lowered brows and unsmiling mouth told us he was in a black mood. A knife could have cut the strained atmosphere that caused. Then as swiftly as it appeared, like sun shining through dark clouds after a rainy day, he changed back into his smiling self.

Within hours of that change, my mother simply glowed with happiness. I saw the presents he came back with – big bouquets of deep pink roses, small parcels wrapped in silvery paper, usually containing pretty bottles of perfume or maybe a small piece of jewellery. The adult me has named those periods that were repeated over and over again the 'honeymoon times'. All the pain of his blows was pushed to the back of Mum's mind, while the man guilty of inflicting them turned into the person she had fallen in love with.

His warm smiles were turned in my direction as well for he stepped back into the caring stepfather role as easily as if he had never stepped out of it. Lessons and criticisms stopped, replaced by mugs of hot chocolate and the freedom to watch TV with them.

Satisfied both my mother and I were likely to agree to just about anything, he did not waste much time asking me where my paints were.

'Come on, fetch them out! You can paint on my legs today,' he said, ruffling my hair.

I wonder if he knew how I had come to loathe looking at his hairy body, something I tried my best to hide. I tried not to touch his skin when I drew on it with my paintbrush and had to stop myself from cringing visibly each time when by accident, I did so. Though now I understand more of how his mind worked, I realise that of course he knew. I hated how he got his kicks by forcing me to do whatever he told me. The fact that it was something I loathed just gave him satisfaction – he would have seen how much I flinched when I was marched to the shower. He was totally aware of how scared I was of the water stinging my skin and getting in my eyes.

And he knew that I already felt what he was doing was wrong.

What he didn't know was how determined I was not to give in to panic. I remembered then and still do that it was his hands on my shoulders that had held me under that water when I was just five. And his laughter mingled with my mother's as I struggled to breathe that caused my meltdown. If I had not forgotten that, neither had he. Which is why I was so determined I would collapse again. Well, who would want to be mocked for something they couldn't help? At five, I might have expected some kindness but by seven, I knew it was not going to be forthcoming.

My future stepfather was a man of almost entirely inflexible habits so I knew what to expect each time my shower was finished. A large towel would be wrapped around me before he rubbed me down. I tried not to wriggle away when, through the thick fabric, I felt his hands linger on different parts of my body. I might just have stepped out of the shower but his wandering paws made me feel grubbier than when I stepped into it.

'Go and put your pyjamas on and I'll make you a warm drink,' he told me each time. It made me swallow involuntarily for I already knew what was to follow.

Hot chocolate had become part of his evening ritual. That part I liked, the second I did not.

It began with him placing me on his knee for what he called 'a cuddle'. Gradually, it progressed to him moving his body up against mine. I wanted to escape, get off his lap, but as though sensing how I felt, his hand tightened on my hair. This was his far-from-subtle way of reminding me how he nearly pulled it out by the roots. Gritting my teeth, I stayed put as he moved up and down with my face tucked into his shoulder.

The second or third time he repeated that act, he pulled a rug over us.

'Keep you warm,' he said as he bounced steadily underneath me. I could feel him, feel that part that was meant for peeing against my bottom. It grew hard as he rubbed against me, making me want to squirm away from him.

Fear warned, *You upset him and you know what will happen. Do you really want any more bruises? Just grit your teeth and it will soon be over.* Looking back, I'm lucky not to have damaged those teeth for I seemed to have spent much of my childhood gritting them in an effort not to make him lose his temper.

My mother must have known what was happening. I mean, she often came into the room but if she had any thoughts about what he was doing, she kept them to herself. There were even a couple of times when she spoke to him while I was on his lap.

Although I knew that Carl's good moods were never going to last long, the repugnance I felt at what he was doing to me was mixed with relief that he was going through a good-tempered phase. *Another reason to stop me protesting?* I had been there too many times not to know the slightest thing could set him off. An imaginary insult, disregarding his wishes or just that he had got out of bed on the wrong side. Once I saw that darkness return, I did my best to make myself invisible as, quaking with fear, I tiptoed around the house. But until then, he ceased shouting at me for what he considered my numerous misdemeanors. Even better, he stopped both forcing lessons on me and interrogating me on what I had learnt at school the moment I walked through the door.

He even stopped making comments about my eating habits, though I was aware that they were being watched carefully.

*   *   *

When I separated my vegetables into small individual piles, I could feel his eyes on me. I felt his disapproval at my portion of red meat always being well done. Not that my mother did that out of kindness, more because she didn't want me throwing up. I had heard him say more than once that she was just pandering to me, which was his way of saying she was enabling my habits. Her answer was that she had learnt to tolerate them.

I always had a sense of foreboding that one day, he would do more than just voice his disapproval. Though when he was in a good mood, Mum didn't seem to care how I ate. She was just happy that there was peace in the house. Not to mention being presented with those little gifts of flowers and perfume.

The school was also fairly easy-going. My mother had explained some of my 'quirks', as I prefer to call them, to the head teacher when I first started there. Not, I think now for my sake, but because she didn't want a phone call informing her that I had just had a meltdown and upset the whole class. Now that she would have found really embarrassing. Plus, she might have worried just what I might tell them when I was in that state. She also told the headmistress that she had consulted a doctor about my habits and his response was that there was nothing to be concerned about.

Well, that's the story she told Carl – another one of her lies. It was *her mother* who had done that. I had heard Gran telling Mum exactly what it was the doctor had said. His advice was there are children who are sensory sensitive and for them, routine is very important. They get confused, even upset, with too many changes. The word 'autism' was not mentioned, nor was there any suggestion of my being assessed. Even in the nineties, it was not something that all doctors were aware of. But at least he understood sensory processing problems, which was a bonus.

He did admit, my grandmother told her, that he didn't understand what caused it, but as long as the right allowances were made, there was nothing much to worry about.

'So, you're telling me that she's not going to grow out of it?' snapped Mum when that was explained to her.

'Now, Betty, that's enough! It's not much of a problem now, is it?'

Not to Gran perhaps.

I once heard Mum ranting about it to my dad, asking him if 'idiot' behaviour ran in his family. His answer was that I was hardly an idiot just because I had some rather odd ways. Then he picked up the newspaper and held it high above his head, letting her know that all conversation on the matter was over.

That was then, or rather before Carl came into our lives.

If I have anything to be grateful for regarding my genes, it is that I'm so low on the spectrum. I do have empathy and a sense of humour, thank goodness. I shudder to think what might have happened to me, had I been just a tiny bit higher on it. Even if my body had survived my childhood, I doubt my mind would have. And no one would have been able to tell why.

Now, there's a frightening thought.

Chapter 21

I was right in thinking that Carl didn't want to put up with my eating habits any longer. He had the same way of thinking as a man who would punish his son for being left-handed: his home had to be perfect and that included the people who lived in it.

Unfortunately for me, I had no warning of just what he had planned.

I had arrived back from Gran's just after five to be greeted not by him, but my mother, wearing one of her pretty dresses and smelling of perfume. Fully made up too, I noticed. She certainly seemed in an elated mood. She even gave me a warm smile and asked how my day had been.

'Your stepfather,' as she insisted on calling him, 'is cooking for us tonight. That makes a change, doesn't it?'

As I had hardly ever seen him help with any of the domestic duties, I wondered just what he was up to.

'Why?' I asked.

'Because he wants to do something nice for us, Emily, and we have something to celebrate which involves you as well. So, he wants us to tell you about it once we are all sitting down.'

I had a premonition then that this was not going to be the pleasant evening she was trying to say it was. All right, it was Carl who had planned everything but then, hard as it is even to accept all these years later, she already knew what he was up to.

Let's just say he must have had a load of fun putting together that menu. No wonder he busied himself in the kitchen for the first and only time.

I watched my mother as in between laying the table and opening a bottle of red wine *to allow it to breathe*, she busied herself in running back and forth to the kitchen to see if he needed any help.

'You go and tidy yourself up,' she told me. 'Your hair could do with a brush and make sure you wash your hands as well.'

I should have smelt a rat, a big stinking one – him cooking and her being nice to me was more than a little unusual. But I was just happy that there was no bad atmosphere and that she was being so friendly. At that age I was easily won over all right! So, trustingly, off I went to tidy myself, wondering what the surprise that I was to be included in was going to be.

When I came back, the kitchen door swung open, letting out the aroma of my least favourite smell – meat cooking.

Big smile from him as well, they certainly were a happy pair that evening. 'A little celebration,' he told me as he crossed the room to pour them both a drink.

'Gin and tonic, darling,' he murmured, passing her a glass, and 'Orange juice for you, Emily,' he added to my surprise. I was not usually – well, ever – included in their evening drinks ritual.

'Cheers, both of you,' he said with another baring of teeth as he flashed that broad smile of his in my direction.

I stood there patiently waiting to be told just what we were celebrating. And I knew not to ask; they would tell me when they were ready.

'Well, Emily, I'm sure you must be beside yourself with curiosity about what we have to tell you, aren't you?'

'Yes,' I admitted, forcing myself to smile back at him.

'What we want to say is that your mother has agreed to marry me and you are to be our bridesmaid. Great news, isn't it? It means I really will be your stepdad then. Now, what do you think of that?'

Better not tell him, muttered Fear.

'When will it be?' I managed to ask, trying my hardest to look happy.

'Oh, in about six weeks, so there are lots of plans to make. And there are dresses for you and your mother to buy. So, what have you got to say, Emily?'

'Sounds really good,' I replied, forcing another smile on my face, though my suddenly weak legs refused to carry me over to Mum and give her a hug, which no doubt might have been expected.

What I really wanted was to run out of the room, grab a pillow and scream into it.

Hadn't I hoped that every time I had heard their rows and the sounds of him hitting her that she would throw him out? Just seeing the radiant expression on my mother's

face that evening told me there was no chance of that happening. Any hopes I might have had died in that room that
night. He was to remain in my life, that was the uncomfortable truth, and the truth jangled at my nerves, squeezing
my stomach muscles.

Marriage, I was certain, would give him even more
power over my life if that were possible.

And I was just about to find out that I was right.

Through the fuzz in my brain I heard that they planned to
look for a house – 'Big enough if we add to our family,' Carl
said with a smirk, which was his way of letting me know that
they planned to have more children. Then another thought
struck me: *Please don't let it be far away from here.*

*Surely he would not move us away from everyone we
knew?*

'Where will it be?' I asked, trying to look interested
although that sinking feeling in my stomach was growing.

'Oh, not too far from here,' came the answer. 'Just further out of town, we want some outside space. Be good for
you, won't it?'

So, why did I have a feeling then that the move was part
of Carl's larger plan? On that evening, I couldn't see what
it was but somehow I knew he had formulated one.

'Now, the meal needs some of my attention. No, my
darling, you two stay put,' he told Mum as she made a
move to follow him into the kitchen. 'I'll bring everything
in when it's ready.'

If I wondered what he had cooked, I was soon to find
out when he carried in a huge platter of rare meat and a

bowl full of mixed vegetables. I saw straight away that they would be impossible for me to sort into different colours, though that was nothing like as bad as the meat.

Just looking at it sitting in its pink-tinged juices made my stomach churn and the bile started to rise in my throat. The thought of eating it was enough to send shivers down my spine. If I put one piece of it in my mouth, I would vomit it up straight away. I felt Carl's eyes on me and looking up, I knew he was totally aware of what I was going through.

End of nice stepfather role all right! I wonder now what dark thoughts went through his head when he decided to cook a meal that would make a seven-year-old child feel physically sick.

I looked across at my mother – she understood, didn't she? No help was to come from her, I realised, when she studiously avoided my gaze.

'Mum,' I whispered, trying desperately to get her attention, 'you know I can't eat that!'

'You'll have to try, Emily. Carl cooked this especially for us.'

Well, that was clear all right! He cooked it specially to show me up, more like it.

'I can't,' I said, swallowing down the bitter-tasting bile making its way up my throat again.

Carl said nothing, just stood there, and without looking at him, I could feel his glare burning into my skin.

Without uttering a sound, he drew my chair from the table, caught me by the back of my neck, pulled me over to the chair and threw me forcibly onto it. Then he moved it firmly right up to the table. I watched with something approaching horror as he leant over the table and speared a piece of meat. He waved it just under my nose, making sure I could smell it. His eyes fixed on mine as he swiftly brought it to my mouth and tried to ram the piece into it.

I couldn't help shutting my mouth so firmly it was as though my jaws had locked themselves tight all on their own – I couldn't open them if I tried. Not that he was about to give up: he gripped my jaw and tried to force it open while holding the blood-flecked meat.

'Open your mouth, Emily, or I'll open it for you.'

But I couldn't, my jaw really had locked tightly shut.

His face was filled with anger, those grey eyes of his burning into me, but the more scared I became, the more my mouth refused to open. Giving up, he pulled me from the chair, his arm raised, and I felt the cold, sharp skin of his hand connecting hard against my jaw. As I tasted the metallic sting of blood inside my mouth, I knew the monster in him was fully awake.

Another thump, this time to my head, and I saw stars as I fell to the floor.

He gripped my arm and pulled me up.

'Go to your room and stay out of my sight!' he hissed.

A command that was easy to obey as I staggered along the corridor, praying he would not come after me. I managed to open the door and throw myself onto the bed before finally blacking out.

When I came to, it was to find my mother, a worried expression on her face, sitting on the end of my bed. My face was throbbing, my head ached, and all I wanted was to close my eyes and drift off into unconsciousness again.

'Here,' she said and placed a freezing-cold towel on the side of my face that he had hit. 'Ice will help get rid of the swelling,' she told me matter-of-factly. 'Now, take these,' she added, placing two painkillers in my hand and passing me a glass of water.

It hurt even to open my mouth wide enough to swallow them and gulp down the water to get them down.

'He's sorry he hit you,' she said, still in that same tone.

Not 'How *dare* he touch my daughter, I'm leaving the bastard! The wedding is off!' Oh no, nothing like that. Her concern was that he had nearly knocked me out and there was only so much damage to me that she could cover up.

Yes, sorry he had not taken off his rings, I suspected. My jaw was bruised – in fact, so bruised and swollen, I had to be kept off school.

Sorry she had to fob off her mother from visiting me when she was told I was unwell?

Sorry she had to tell the same story to my dad?

I wonder now if she had any doubts on entering that marriage. She must have seen how her life would change, surely? If she did, she had firmly pushed them away.

And Carl? Well, he apologised for what he had done. Told me he only wanted to help me rid myself of those habits of mine, that he was concerned that when I was older, people would mock me.

I didn't believe one word of it.

Chapter 22

For some time before the wedding was announced, I had come to realise that it was not only me who Carl exercised his power over, it was my mother as well. Gone was the bossy, sharp-tongued woman I had known ever since I could remember. In her place was someone who agreed with everything he said and just about everything he did – which included him making my life hell. It was as though he had taken the mother I knew and replaced her with his own creation, one who no longer had any opinions of her own.

I still don't know how he managed it, for it hardly took him long to control how Mum spent her time, who she was able to see, and I suspect, even what she thought. Not only that, but since he moved in, Carl had steadily managed to put a distance between us and my mother's family. There were those unsubtle verbal digs aimed at them. He said her sisters and their husbands were jealous of us, that Gran disapproved of her, and was constantly reminding her of his belief that no matter how hard he tried in bringing presents for the children and flowers, chocolates and beers for the adults, they made no effort to accept him as part of their family.

He even suggested that Mum was the least favourite one, frequently reporting snide remarks about her that he claimed to have overheard at the family get togethers. Were they true? I doubt it – it was just his way of trying to make her suspicious and distrust her family.

And finally, after she agreed to marry him, he said he hoped she knew just how much he was looking forward to the wedding: 'It means we three will be a proper family.'

Just goes to show how little he knew about the meaning of the word.

* * *

Even though Carl had put doubts in my mother's mind about the loyalty of her sisters, she still continued to arrange to go to those monthly lunches with them. And what do you know? They nearly always fell on a day when he was suddenly free from work: 'Oh, just say you can't make it today,' he told her gaily when he turned up from his business, saying he had finished unexpectedly early. 'I'll take you out somewhere nice. You'd like that, wouldn't you?' And a kiss was planted on her cheek.

The first time he did it, I saw a flash of annoyance cross her face. *She's going to say she's going anyhow*, I thought then. But, oh no, she quickly smiled back at him and said she would give her sisters a ring to cancel and hoped they would understand.

'Darling, we have a few minutes before we need to leave so you have time to change and put some lipstick on,' he said.

Well, that was telling her, I thought. *I mean, she was already wearing make-up and dressed for lunch with her mum and sisters, wasn't she?*

But Carl didn't do casual and relaxed, and he hated the flat shoes she always wore for these gatherings. 'Heels are much more feminine,' I had heard him say on more than one occasion. Followed by, 'And let's face it, your sisters have let themselves go a bit, haven't they?' before, with a smile, he patted her on her still-slim behind.

I could just imagine what my aunts would have said if their husbands had told them to change. Far less what their fate would have been if a remark like 'You've let yourself go' was mentioned. But, Mum seemed to think it was flattering that he took such an interest in her appearance. He had certainly managed to change it quite a bit. No more lounging around the house in tracksuits for her anymore, or sitting down for dinner without a face full of make-up.

After succeeding the first time, it was an act he seemed to take enjoyment in repeating.

'Right,' she would say each time, 'I won't be long.' A few minutes later she was back wearing a tight clingy dress, her feet pushed into high-heeled shoes and her subtle pink lipstick replaced by a vivid red one.

'That's better,' was his usual comment as he looked her up and down. Then, taking her arm, he would open the door and off they went. At least I had some peace to read my latest book from the library, all about the Greek gods.

After that first time when I saw the flash of annoyance when he bounced in, telling her to cancel her lunch, those subsequent times she responded differently and it seemed that her annoyance was slowly being replaced by acceptance. Even at my young age, I thought I recognised an approaching defeated air about her.

'My sisters were fine about it,' was all she said after each phone call. 'They understand.'

She was right there, they probably did.

From the snippets I overheard after the third time it happened, and the odd comment my cousin Ben made to me, it seemed they were not in the least bit fooled by those last-minute cancellations.

They understood all right, just not in the way she hoped for.

* * *

Once Carl had controlled the amount of times Mum saw her sisters and visited her mother, he must have decided it was essential to tackle those family lunches too. He knew they were something both Mum and I had always looked forward to. When their relationship was new, I had heard her tell him it had been a family tradition for many years. In fact, before he came into our lives, apart from when I had succumbed to a few childhood ailments, we never missed one.

Nevertheless, it was a tradition he was determined to break. He told her that now they were getting married, he wanted us to spend more time together doing our own family things. Not that we seemed to know what he had planned until the last minute. Were we going to the family or not seemed to be a question she was too frightened to ask. Instead, she waited until he told her his plans, which was usually less than an hour before we were due to be there. Then it would be yet another phone call cancelling the arrangements. I would hear her trying to make it sound as though a surprise outing was romantic, while I just swallowed my disappointment.

They weren't even married yet and he was in full control, just how much worse could it get once that knot was tied? Already he was steadily getting what he wanted – my mother completely dependent on him, and me becoming more and more isolated with no one left to confide in. Fear might be able to control a small child, but what about an older one? Something that the adult me thinks he must have thought about round about then. Later, when I became a teenager and found out what his plan for my future really was, his earlier actions became as clear as day. Right from the start, he had a master plan and our lives were all mapped out long before he asked my mother to marry him.

All I understood during those earlier years was that I missed my old life so much. Those carefree days with my cousins and the special times I spent with my grandmother when I had felt both loved and lovable. Piece by piece, the part of my life that had given me such stability was fast disappearing. I can remember now the loneliness of those Saturdays when yet another excuse had been made to turn down an invitation to a family get together.

'Oh dear, I had something special planned for us,' was Carl's usual excuse when he saw Mum and I getting ready. Not that he ever made any arrangements to include me. He just said, 'Now you can help your mother by washing the breakfast dishes, can't you? And when you're done, I suggest you catch up on your homework, Emily.' Those would always be his last words to me before he swept my mother through the door.

Where was the 'We will do things as a family' idea? I wondered after they had swanned out of the house yet again, leaving me alone.

In a way, apart from feeling both angry and miserable at not getting to see the family once more, even though I would be alone for most of the day, it was still a relief when they had gone. While I washed the breakfast dishes I thought about everyone else in my family getting food, drink and themselves ready for the get together. At least on my own I had peace to immerse myself in my own thoughts. When it was just the three of us at home after Carl had persuaded Mum to turn down yet another invitation, it was hard not to show my resentment. And any show of objecting to his decisions did not go down well – it wouldn't take him long to find something to punish me for.

Throughout those lonely days my mind was filled with images of what was taking place without me. I could see my cousins laying the long table and I wondered which one had been delegated to do my task and put out the cushions. My uncles would be busying themselves with getting the coals just the right heat for grilling, while their wives carried out those heaped plates of food. As the day progressed, I thought of my cousins kicking the ball round and Ben giving someone else that high five when a goal was scored.

It was when I let my mind stray to how Gran would have sorted out my food and her smile, so full of love as she gave it to me, that tears pricked my eyes – I just wanted those days back so much. Without my family, I no longer felt I was the special little girl my gran had repeatedly told me I was over the years. In such a short time I had gone from being the much-loved youngest cousin to the girl no one wanted.

Well, that's who I was, wasn't I? Lily didn't seem to want me, nor did my mother. As for my father – well, I wanted to believe he did, but then how many times had my mother told me that it was only because of the law that he spent any time with me? *So, let's face it*, my nasty little inner voice said, *he doesn't want you either. Not now he has another little girl to love, one who won't have your embarrassing eating habits or any of your other odd ways.*

There's nothing like wallowing in self-pity to see the world collapsing all around is you, is there?

My excuse for that little girl I was then was she was still only seven and those small drops of poison were dropped into her ears on a very regular basis. The saddest thing was that she truly believed all of it. Her confidence began to disappear, she thought all she did was annoy and irritate all the people around her, and so she closed herself off from her school friends, telling them she wanted to be left alone.

Even the fact that the teachers kept praising her school-work failed to reassure her. Hadn't Carl told her they were just being kind because she was different?

'And what will happen to you when you grow up?' he kept saying. 'You're not going to find being an adult easy, are you? Who's going to want to give you a job? So, you'd better listen to me – I only hit you to make you realise that.'

And the little girl I had once been had no choice but to believe him.

Chapter 23

During the week, I was still able to see Gran although it was never long enough. The moment I heard that phone ring to signal that I was to go home, I would clench my fists so hard, my nails left small red crescents on my palms. My gran was always careful not to mention what was planned for the weekend or tell me about the previous one, if I had not been there. I assume because she had got wise to Carl's manipulations and didn't want to build my hopes up only to see them dashed at the last minute. Without saying anything, she must have understood how disappointed I would have been each time he insisted that our acceptance was cancelled – she never asked me what we did instead either.

Did she know they left me in the flat alone?

I don't know. She never asked, perhaps guessing that I had gradually been programmed to lie about what went on in our home. I'm sure she understood that for most of the week I hoped that Carl would not stop us coming for lunch and it must have made her angry when she realised by the timing of her daughter's phone call that he had left it until the last minute to tell us. She would have recognised it was yet another of his power games.

I had learnt through Ben that our turning down invitations really concerned not just my gran but everyone else in our family; they were not happy about my situation either.

'They worry about you, Emily,' my cousin told me nearly every time he took me home. He couldn't stop himself from running Carl down either, not mincing his words when he recounted just what the family thought of him now: 'That man of your mum's is such a controlling prick!' he declared angrily. 'That's what my dad thinks anyway and so do I.'

It was clear from that comment and other snippets he told me that the initial good impression Carl had made when he was first introduced to the family had worn well and truly thin. Not one of them trusted him, especially since I had had that meltdown.

'And none of us think he's kind to you or your mother,' Ben told me on another of our journeys home. 'You've both changed since he arrived. I mean, your mum used to be a bit of a bitch really, like always bossing your dad around, but now she's meek as a lamb. She never leaves his side when you do turn up, so what's he done to you both?' His eyes scanned my face as he said this, perhaps trying to fathom out what my response would be.

Each time he brought it up, I wanted to burrow my face into his shoulder, sob loudly and tell him what was happening. Maybe if he had been a few years older I would have, but he was still at school. And anything I told him would be repeated to his father. How could I be certain that the whole family thought the same way about Carl as Ben did?

After all, they were nice enough about him when we did meet.

'That's because we don't want to stop seeing you,' was Ben's explanation when I put it to him.

Anyhow, Fear was hardly quiet during those exchanges, even interrupting my cousin more than once: *He'll say you're making it all up, won't he? And then Carl will punish you* was an oft-repeated remark blocking out some of Ben's conversation.

Then I heard Ben saying that the family really wanted me to visit more: 'Well, the truth is they want to keep an eye on you. That's why they're careful not to do or say anything which might give him a reason for you not to come at all. They're aware that he looks down on us, thinks we're country bumpkins. That's rich, isn't it, coming from a bloke who's moved into your mother's flat! Anyhow, what is it he does for a living? That's what everyone is curious about.'

'I don't know,' was the answer I gave, for that was the truth then and is remarkably still the truth today.

All I'd ever heard him mention were some property deals he was taking care of. When I repeated that to the curious Ben, he burst out laughing.

'That's what he told my dad too. What?! And he's not moved you both into a nice big swanky house? I don't believe that for one single minute! Still, he never seems short of money, does he?'

I didn't have any idea about that either. Just that there were times when there seemed to be plenty of money around and other times when his mood turned even blacker and he told Mum and I that we had to spend carefully for a while.

Most times when he took me home, Ben would try and reassure me that I could always talk to him. His other piece of advice was, 'Just don't ever let him change you, Emily.'

As if I had any choice in the matter.

Chapter 24

What had I told you about Carl? That he wanted everything he owned to be perfect. The next stage of his turning us into puppets who only danced to his tune was dictating what we wore. He had already managed to change how my mother dressed and now he turned his attention to me. Not that he didn't appear to disguise it so well. To any unsuspecting person, his sending Mum out with me to purchase a completely new wardrobe might have been seen as an act of generosity and caring. And I might have gone along with that thought, had I been given any choice in the matter.

Not only did I have no choice, neither did my mother.

He had written a list of the clothes and shoes he wanted her to buy for me. It was he who decided on the colours of each item, not to mention the exact style of shoes. No more dungarees and brightly coloured T-shirts for me – *'too boyish,'* he insisted. In fact, no brightly coloured *anything* was specified. My reds and bright yellows were taken to the charity shop. Sensible navy-blue skirts and grey or dark blue jumpers were prescribed for winter – *'More ladylike'*. Even worse were the black lace-up shoes he said were *'good for her feet'*, although everyone else was wearing slip-ons – *'Their parents don't care if they damage their feet'*. Later, I would think back and wonder why he insisted on Mum squeezing her feet into stilettos. His choice of my summer clothes – stiff cotton dresses in the darkest shades he could find (*'They suit you'*) – was no better.

They didn't.

Clumpy dark brown sandals replaced the black lace-ups.

He didn't approve of the *'female sex'* as he put it wearing trousers or shorts. The only concession he made here was that I could don them when cycling.

Once my new clothes were hanging up neatly, he announced that he had arranged something else for both of us – new hairstyles. In Mum's case a photo of the actress Kim Novak was dangled in front of her. Not that I knew who she was, just that I saw little resemblance between her and my mother.

'You could look like that,' I heard him say, 'so I've made an appointment for you to have your hair lightened and cut into a chic bob. You will look just wonderful, I know you will.

'What do you think, Emily?' he asked, waving the photo in front of my face.

Not that he wanted my opinion, he just wanted me to agree with him.

'She's very pretty,' was all I could think of to say.

'And so is your mother!' he snapped.

I thought it would take more than a new hairstyle to work that kind of magic. Surely Carl did not see her as that pretty woman's double? I mean, my mum was attractive, but looked nothing like the photo.

But he continued with his instructions: 'I've arranged for you to have a makeover as well once your hair is done – facial, nails, the works!' His face beamed as he told her, basking in his own, as he saw it, generosity. Good thing he was too snobbish to read the tabloids, or he might have read all about the wonders of plastic surgery. I hate to think how she might have finished up, had he decided she needed a few nips and tucks.

A couple of days later when Ben brought me home, there was my makeover mother. Not only had she had a new hairstyle – a short, pale blonde bob with lots of high-lights – her nails were a perfect pink and her lips seemed plumper, more glossy. Her eyelashes also seemed to have grown twice as long since breakfast and her eyebrows were plucked into a neat arch which gave her a permanent faintly enquiring look.

'What do you think?' she asked, flapping her manicured hands in front of me.

'Like the colour of your hair, Mum, you look nice,' was all I could manage.

'Yes, her new hairdresser's good – my friends' wives all go there,' Carl said with a smirk that bothered me. With a sinking feeling, I guessed what his next words were going to be: 'And you're next for your treat, Emily. I've booked you in there for a professional hairstyle too. Now, what do you say to that?'

Well, I had to say thank you, didn't I? The truth was the idea of a stranger touching my hair absolutely terrified me.

I had wavy hair and when it was not tied back, it fell to my shoulders. It was Aunt Lizzy who trimmed it every so often. She and my gran always remarked on how pretty it was, even though it took ages to wash and brush. Both of them understood my sensory processing problems and that the slightest tug could cause me real pain – but would the hairdresser?

Hardly, I thought.

Talk about being caught between a rock and a hard place! Saying I didn't want my hair done would result in a painful punishment, because even Carl could not drag a protesting seven-year-old into a hair salon against her wishes.

A hairdresser who did not understand my condition would also hurt me though.

But not as bad as he will, said Fear. *Best grit your teeth and grin and bear it!*

* * *

Saturday morning, up I got and dressed in one of those new outfits that I so disliked. *Best to please him*, I told myself as I pulled on the dark skirt and jumper. It was Carl, not my mother, who was taking me to the hairdresser. I wondered how he was going to tell her to style it – I just hoped it would not be like Mum's.

The moment I walked into the busy salon my ears were attacked by the cacophony of background music, hairdryers and conversation. Glancing around nervously, the first thing my eyes rested on were all those pairs of large, shiny scissors. They seemed to be everywhere – in the hands of the stylists, poking out of plastic containers and sticking out of half-open drawers. Just the thought of cold metal touching my head was almost enough to bring on a panic attack, as was the second thing I noticed – washbasins, where water gushed over the heads of people leaning backwards over them. I froze, staring in horror at this procedure.

To my utmost relief, Carl just told the assistant to spray my hair damp enough to cut it, as it was clean. I doubt if that was for my sake, more likely to stop him being embarrassed at my having a complete meltdown. Still, whatever the reason, I felt grateful.

'Just a bit of a trim?' asked the hairdresser, holding my long wavy hair in her hand. 'How do you want it?' she asked me.

'Short,' replied Carl, before I had a chance to say anything.

'How short, sir? She has such lovely hair. How about I neaten it up a little, keep some of the length?'

'No, I want it cut like this,' he said and out came another embarrassing photo of the actress Audrey Hepburn when she was young. Again, she was not a name I recognised, nor did the stylist when he told her. But whoever she was,

I was embarrassed because with her delicate elfin features, there was no way I resembled her.

'Ah, the urchin look,' she said, but I heard the doubt in her voice.

Still, it was he who was paying, but I could tell she didn't think it a good idea any more than I did.

I have to tell you that both back then and right up until today, short hair doesn't suit me. And I still don't have one feature that resembles the waif-like Hepburn.

'Now, Emily,' Carl said to me in the warm voice he used only in public, his fingers fidgeting with his rings, 'you'll be a good girl, won't you?' He smiled as he saw my gaze was riveted on his hands. Right on cue, he gave the signet ring a harder twist and I gulped as that familiar icy fear flooded me.

'Yes,' was all I managed to say.

I grabbed both arms of the chair as the hairdresser examined me critically in the mirror. Out came the spray that wetted my hair before she picked up those long, shining scissors. Before she cut off one lock, I was completely stiffened with fright from just sitting there. Already I could feel the blades snickering away and imagined my dark locks laying in clumps on the floor. I'm sure she thought I was shaking at the thought of losing my hair, not the fact that I could hardly bear the feel of her hands or the sound of those cold, metal scissors snipping away.

Finally, the hairdryer was switched on and hot air blasted on my neck while the stylist's fingers ran through my hair as she styled the blow-dry. I kept thinking how annoyed my gran would be when she saw how short my hair was now. Once the stylist had finished, a carefully angled mirror showed me how it looked at the back, although I was still glancing in dismay at my reflection in the front one. She had done the best she could, giving me a choppy fringe and a few soft wisps to frame my face.

All I could see was how different I looked, and not in a good way. My face looked rounder, my nose larger. Even at seven, I knew instinctively that it did not suit me.

Not that Carl agreed when he walked in.

'Very stylish,' he said, giving the stylist a large tip and a beaming smile.

'Pleased?' he asked when we were outside.

'Yes,' I replied, forcing a smile on my face.

I was learning.

Chapter 25

Since my future stepfather had chosen a family get together to announce that there was to be a wedding, our lives had been a constant flurry of activity.

'Got something to tell you all,' he said proudly, tapping his glass to get everyone's attention. 'Betty has agreed to marry me and I feel that I'm the luckiest man alive.'

Meanwhile, my mother, all pink-cheeked and coy smiles, flashed her engagement ring, a diamond set in white gold, for everyone to admire.

The men shook his hand and the women congratulated Mum with hugs and kisses. And my gran tried her hardest to look pleased for them, but I could tell she wasn't.

Once the announcement was out of the way, my mother went shopping with her sisters in search not just for the right dress for her, but for her two bridesmaids: one of my young cousins and myself. She had decided on a white wedding. Now you might think this was hardly appropriate. Especially as I had recently learnt that my birth parents were never actually married, which is why she and Carl could make their vows in church. But still, as I was going to be a bridesmaid and she had been living with him for nearly three years, you would have thought that at least she might have chosen a cream dress. But no, she wanted it all white. And when I say *all* white, she meant *everything* white – bridesmaids' dresses, flowers, shoes and anything else she could possibly think of.

* * *

I'm sure everyone must have breathed a sigh of relief when the wedding was finally arranged. They could see an end to traipsing round shops, looking at pictures of wedding cakes of all designs and sizes, and the endless talk about Mum's diet. At least the date had been settled, the church booked, which only left Carl to sort one thing out – a suitable venue to hold the reception.

One thing I find very characteristic of my stepdad was the actual date of it. He had circled it in for the day after his birthday, August Bank Holiday Monday. I guess it was his way of saying how special he was.

Why not have it on the Saturday? I thought.

When my mother asked the same question, he replied haughtily, 'Only plebs get married on a Saturday.' He wanted two parties in two days, with him being the centre of attention at them both.

The one good thing about it all was that I was getting to see Mum's family a lot more again. They were forever planning together, either with them calling round to our home or we were going over to theirs. As it was all to do with the wedding, Carl could hardly object. I especially loved it when it was just Mum and I visiting Gran's and her sisters came over to join us all. Pots of tea were made, Gran's freshly baked scones perfumed the air and we ate them warm with whipped cream and strawberry jam, except of course my mother – 'Got to look after my waistline'. Naturally, the whole conversation was about the coming event and how her dress had to be taken in because of her drastic diet of no carbs and certainly no sugar.

'So, where are you going for a honeymoon?' Gran asked – a question that had been running through my head ever since I had been told the date of the wedding.

I knew what a honeymoon was – it was where a newly married couple went away for at least two weeks to some exotic country. While they were away, I would have to stay with my gran and have those weekends with my cousins. I held my breath, waiting for Mum to tell her that they were going to France or Italy for two weeks, even three.

A hope that died just as soon as she spoke.

'We've decided not to have one,' she said. 'It's a joint decision,' she added firmly, though I noticed the tell-tale flush on her cheeks rather betrayed her embarrassment. 'It's just that Carl wants us to move into a house as soon as we can and we are putting the money aside for that.'

'And where is he now? You said he was looking at some venues.'

'Yes, he is. He said he wants to make sure we have the right one. He's already talked to a firm of caterers and he's arranging the cake. He's hardly letting me do anything.'

'Well, if you two are putting money aside, why don't you have the reception at our houses?' Aunt Lizzy suggested. 'There's so much room between them, that would save you an awful lot. As long as you got in some help, we could all muck in, sorting out and preparing the food.'

'I don't know what Carl has arranged,' my mother said hesitantly.

'Well, tell him about our offer before he signs anything.'

* * *

When Mum broached the subject with him, Carl turned it down with a burst of derisory laughter – 'I don't think so, Betty! Just think what it would be like. Kids running wild and the men staying at the barbecue, drinking beer out of cans while they talk nonstop about their only interest – football. Not to mention how your mother and your sisters will spend the whole time prattling on about some bit of gossip. I can just see it now.

'Dear me, if that's not just one of the worst ideas you've ever come up with! It's certainly not what I have in mind and I really can't think you have either.'

Again, his sarcastic laughter rang out.

This time my mother did not join in. It was not often I saw her looking angry at anything Carl did or said, but there was no mistaking her reaction. Her face froze without even a glimmer of a smile and was set in anger. A muscle in her cheek started to twitch.

Had he forgotten this was her family he had just ridiculed?

Seeing her response, he patted her on the knee. 'Oh, look, I know it was kind of your family to offer, don't think I'm not grateful. I just want the very best for you, Betty – you deserve it.' This comment finally brought the beginnings of a smile back to her face. 'We might not be going on a honeymoon, but we're not cutting costs on our wedding. Isn't that what you want as well, a really smart affair that everyone will still remember for years?'

Of course, she folded and agreed with him. Which is why, between them, they worked out a compromise: Mum would ask her family to throw a birthday party for Carl at their homes on the Sunday instead. An afternoon affair, he explained, where everyone could have fun and then they would have the more formal wedding the following day.

I wished I could have stuffed my fingers in my ears when they got to the next part of their conversation – where they were going to sleep after the party.

'You know it's bad luck not to have separate rooms before the wedding,' I heard Carl say, giving her one of those winks before his hand slid around her waist. Her response was to giggle and snuggle up to him.

'Guess we'll just have to risk it,' she said, giggling even more.

Personally, I thought marrying him was the risk, but I kept that thought along with many others well and truly to myself.

I wished they would leave those little intimate displays until they were out of my sight. To say they were embarrassing was an understatement. Not that I knew what went on in the bedroom, apart from the times he hit her. I guessed it must have been something like touching each other all over, because I knew he enjoyed that, didn't I? Enough to make me shudder at the thought that this was something my mother *liked* him doing.

I did wonder then why he wanted a birthday party as well as a wedding over the same bank holiday weekend. After all, it would be the same people going to both. Now as I think back to that time, I have a suspicion that he wanted everyone to compare the reception he had arranged to the party Mum's family had thrown for him. It was the first time he had asked if it was OK to invite a few of his friends, or rather men he did business with and their wives. And yes, they would be coming to the wedding as well so it would be them he would want to impress.

* * *

Considering it was approaching autumn, we were having what Carl called 'an Indian summer'. Blue cloudless skies and golden rays of sunshine promised us a rain-free and extremely hot bank holiday weekend. That meant we would all be outside for the birthday party and I would be free to spend time with my cousins.

Except for the pile of presents placed in front of Carl, the raised glasses and the rendition of 'Happy Birthday' sung at the tops of their voices, the celebration was more or less the same as all the other family get togethers. I might not have enjoyed singing 'Happy Birthday', but 'For He's a

Jolly Good Fellow' really made me cringe, although I was enjoying myself playing ball and chatting to my cousin Ben, who had refused to join in any of the singing. He made sure to spend some time with me and was tactful not to mention again my new look in clothes and hairstyle. I will never forget the look of dismay on Gran's face when she first saw it, which she quickly replaced with a smile as she told me how nice it looked.

Not often I had caught my gran out in a lie, but that was definitely one.

I had also noticed Ben's shocked look when I walked in the first time after my 'makeover'. His eyes went up and down my navy-blue outfit as well, before coming to rest on those clumpy black lace-up shoes, but still, he said nothing for which I was grateful. His tact ran out, however, when he spotted the puffiness around my eye: 'So, Sprat, what happened to your eye?' The truth was that this time I really had walked into a cupboard door – it must have been the only injury I had ever given myself.

I saw that the words 'cupboard door' did not impress – it was soon clear that Ben didn't believe me.

'Walked into a cupboard door! Oh, come on now, that's an old one, isn't it?' he said, holding my gaze.

'I really did, promise.'

'All right, Sprat, *this time* it was an accident,' was his reply with emphasis. 'Is it true that Carl hasn't invited one member of his family to the wedding?' he continued. 'Strange, that. My dad says he's just got business connections on his list of guests, really weird. Anyhow, how are you feeling about tomorrow?' he asked, obviously deciding to change the subject.

'Don't like my dress much,' I answered, thinking of that white, wide-skirted bridesmaid's outfit hanging up on the side of my wardrobe.

'Why? What's wrong with it?'

'It scratches and makes me look like a huge meringue,' I answered with a grin.

'You know what I mean, though, don't you? How do you feel about him becoming your stepdad?' he persisted.

'Can't see it making much difference,' I replied matter-of-factly. That was more or less the truth – I was pretty sure once that ring was on Mum's finger, I was stuck with him and my life wasn't going to improve.

'Well, you know I'm always here for you, don't you?' he said, giving my shoulder a reassuring squeeze as I smiled up at him. Then I realised that something behind me had caught his eye. Just as I started to turn my head to see what it was, he grabbed my arm. 'Don't look now, your stepdad's watching us,' he said, 'and he doesn't look too happy either. Just turn around slowly and see for yourself.'

Ben was right, for out of the corner of my eye I could see, even from where we were standing, that Carl was far from pleased about the two of us chatting. Had we been any closer, he would have used some excuse to beckon me over. But he wasn't, and he could hardly call out to me in front of his fancy friends, so I ignored him, which did not stop my stomach from clenching.

He's going to get angry and that's never good, Fear muttered.

Shivers ran down my spine as I pictured him making some excuse to punish me. Because that's what he did, even when I'd done nothing wrong.

He won't this time, said the voice of Reason. *He won't want you having any bruises tomorrow, now will he?*

So, listening to Reason, I made myself relax.

'You're scared of him, aren't you?' said Ben, who had been studying me closely.

'Don't be silly, of course I'm not,' I countered.

'Heard you were sick a few weeks ago and you couldn't go to school, so what was so wrong with you that you couldn't have any visitors?'

'Oh, just flu,' I murmured, managing to repeat what my mother had instructed me to say.

'Mmm . . . OK . . . Yes, that was what I was told too,' he replied and I knew he didn't believe me.

Reason was right: not only did Carl not punish me, but that evening, he surprised both Mum and me.

Chapter 26

The day of the wedding, I woke early and looked with disdain at that frothy white dress which was too fully skirted to fit inside the wardrobe. All too soon, I would have to put it on.

It was Aunt Lizzy who arrived after breakfast to help me dress and do my hair. First on went the stiff net underskirt that felt scratchy against my legs and over it went that wide-skirted dress with its tight bodice. My aunt had realised the net would be a problem when she had seen my mother choose the dress and she dug in her handbag and pulled out some very thick white tights and helped me into them; they stopped the worst of the scratching and I smiled gratefully at her. White ballet pumps, the only good thing about Mum's choice of outfits, were removed from their box and my feet slipped into them – at least I could say goodbye to my hideous sensible shoes for one day.

Next up was getting my hair looking the way my mother had said she wanted it – 'An Alice band, a white velvet one,' I had heard Carl say. Not only were my senses tingling with the touch of the underskirt, but he knew anything on my head would be painful for me. To make matters worse, an arrangement of white roses was somehow meant to be stuck into it. It might have worked with long wavy hair, but not my new shorter style.

I'm sure Aunt Lizzy must have been thinking the same thing.

'Don't worry,' she told me. 'I've got that sorted.' And she produced the white velvet Alice band, pinned some white rosebuds on it and slipped it onto my head as carefully as she could. 'Now, don't you look pretty?' she said as she spun me round to face the mirror.

Well, that might have been her opinion, but it really wasn't mine – at least my hair didn't look too bad.

* * *

What can I say about the ceremony? All I remember is a hard seat that made me want to wriggle, a lot of talking by a creepy-looking priest, rings being exchanged, a kiss that somehow managed to look tender, lovely music pealing out, the couple walking down the aisle and me getting in the procession, followed by my cousin Sally, the other bridesmaid.

If people are meant to cry at weddings because they are so moved, I did not see one tear being wiped away on this occasion. I glanced at my gran, but no, a tear- and smile-free face there all right!

Out we all went for photographs – ones of the bride and groom, others of the bride, groom and bridesmaids. Then the whole family . . . On and on they went, until my mother threw her bouquet of white roses, baby's breath and freesias. We then piled into the hired limousine and were off to the reception.

The other bridesmaid had brought a change of clothes with her: a brightly coloured party dress and a pair of pink glittery sandals. 'It's a party, isn't it?' she said when she spotted my envious gaze.

It might have been for her, but it wasn't going to be one for me.

I had already asked if I could bring a change of clothes only to be told no.

I was to remain in my dress as it had cost a lot of money and I wasn't to be so ungrateful.

The reception was held in a huge room attached to a very smart hotel. Music Carl had chosen was being played through the speakers, and waiters bustled around serving drinks and elaborate canapés before we sat down. I was seated on one side of Carl, my mother on the other.

Then came the food: oysters and foie gras for the starters. Judging by the expression on the faces of some of my mother's family, they might have preferred the burgers Carl had mentioned.

Swallowing an oyster for the first time at seven was not a nice experience, I can tell you! It took all my willpower not to spit it out. Luckily, it was a small one that slid down my throat before I could spit it out and it stayed down too. The foie gras wasn't too bad – good thing I had no idea about those force-fed geese when I ate it.

Wine was kept flowing, as were soft drinks. After the main course of poached salmon and summer pudding for dessert, cheese and liqueurs followed. Carl had not stinted himself, that was for sure. When his business friends, wearing their smart suits and wide smiles came over to the top table (not that I was introduced to any of them), I heard them praise his choice of venue and say the meal was wonderful – 'And such wonderful wine pairings!' one of them exclaimed.

Then came the speeches. I could almost feel sorry for Mum's eldest brother, Peter – who no one had seen in years – having to stand up and say how they had welcomed Carl into the family. I was beginning to feel uncomfortable, the net underskirt was scratching and my headband had become heavier, so I missed a lot of it.

Afterwards, the DJ did his bit, tunes from the sixties blared out and couples imitating the teenagers they had been back then were soon shaking and twisting the night away happily.

'Come on, Sprat,' said Ben, suddenly appearing at our table, his hand outstretched to take mine.

'She's too young!' Carl snapped. 'Think you'd better find someone else your own age. She can stay here.'

For a moment Ben looked startled before saying very calmly to Carl, 'All right,' and then, 'See you at school tomorrow, Sprat,' to me before walking off.

And stay there I did – bolt upright, watching all the guests having fun and wishing I was anywhere but there.

Chapter 27

Not long after we had returned home from the reception, Carl disappeared for a few minutes and came back, holding three prettily wrapped packages.

For a moment, I thought they were more presents for him.

But I was wrong.

Two were handed to me and one to my mother.

'Tomorrow is the start of us being a family,' he said. 'So here are my presents to both of you.'

I must say I was a bit dumbstruck at this show of good humour. Plus, I was being handed *two* presents, while my mother was only being given one. Not only that, but with all the preparations for the wedding, Carl had seemed too busy to lay down any new draconian rules, which of course meant I had not been punished for forgetting them. So, he had little reason to try and get round me, which he was known to do after one of his severe beatings.

Also, I was now certain that he disliked my friendship with Ben intensely. I had seen the anger on his face at the birthday party when he had spotted me with my cousin. And all that day I had felt his gaze burning into me whenever I was in his sight. And how about how he had spoken to Ben just a few hours earlier when he asked me to dance? So why was he trying to be so nice to me? It was not like him to put his anger to one side, whatever the reason.

He's up to something, whispered Fear.

'Open that one first,' said Carl, breaking into my thoughts, still with that beaming smile I never trusted fixed firmly on his face. I could feel his eyes boring into me as I undid the gold-coloured string and carefully pulled off the wrapping. Inside was a narrow box and inside that a silver pen.

'Like it?' he asked.

I did, it was just so sleek. I was sure that no one at my school had one as nice as this. As I picked it up and found it fitted snugly into my hand, my suspicions simply melted away.

'Oh yes, I do! It's the best present ever,' I told him, my face breaking into a wide smile of delight.

'Excellent! Now, can you guess what's in the other parcel?'

'A book?' I asked, for the shape told me that it probably was.

'You're warm, but we'll let your mother open hers first, shall we?' he said, while I folded the wrapping paper carefully – he couldn't stand mess.

'Now it's your turn,' he told Mum with one of those winks I hated so much. He no doubt thought he looked sexy; I just thought they made him look creepy.

I watched her take care of her pink nails as she opened her parcel delicately to reveal a dark blue square box.

'Don't just look at it, darling, open it!'

Smiling up at him, she removed the lid and gave a gasp of pleasure. Carl was certainly doing well in that direction.

'Oh, it's so beautiful, Carl!' she sighed as she lifted out a silver bracelet with a single charm, a silver replica of a church, dangling from one of its links. 'I love it, I really love it,' she added, as he moved to her side to fasten it round her wrist.

'Better open your other one now,' Mum told me as she jangled her bracelet so that the church swung back and forth.

Instead of the book I had been expecting inside, the parcel contained something much better: a thick cream-coloured diary, complete with a tiny brass lock.

'Oh, thank you, thank you!' I squealed, holding it tightly to my chest. My face, I'm sure, was bright pink with pleasure as I beamed up at him.

It was something I had wanted for ages. I enjoyed writing. Without someone to confide in, I often had the urge to put down on paper what my thoughts and wishes were. But I would never have dared write them in a notebook – I was far too careful to do that. I knew he went into my room when I was out and on my return, I could see that things had been moved slightly. Occasionally, I could smell his aftershave hanging in the air, which told me he had only just left when he heard me coming through the front door. But now I could write in my diary and then put the lock on. I could share my thoughts and secrets with it – I even had the best pen ever to write in it.

'I saw this in a shop and thought it had your name on it,' said Carl, smiling at my obvious pleasure. 'Well, they both did actually – I've seen you scribbling away. Let's call them early birthday presents. You're going to be eight very soon, aren't you? Now, here's your last little gift. Hold your hand out,' and he dropped a minute brass key into it.

I really can't blame my seven-year-old self for being so gullible. It never entered her head just why he had given her those presents. She was too busy stroking the cover of the diary and thinking how wonderful it was to have a journal where she could write whatever she wanted inside to question why he had done it. Why, in that moment she almost felt a wave of affection for the giver of that diary.

But that was then.

It took nearly four years before she finally learnt the reason; four years of being given a new diary on each of her birthdays. Four years of her confiding to what she thought was her secret friend. You know that expression, 'I wish I could see into your head?' Well, with those diaries in her room, he could. All her thoughts and wishes, who she had spoken to, who were her friends at school, and his biggest worry, what she and Ben talked about.

Everything was in those pages.

The idea of me having a journal was completely his idea, of course. What better way to know everything I thought, felt and planned to do?

What better way to get into my head?

The child I was then had become a reserved little girl. One who had learnt to keep any opinions to herself and never, ever say anything about her home life. Which did not mean her mind did not stop racing. There was so much bottled up inside my younger self for there was no one she dared confide in, no one to share what was really going on and no one to stop her loneliness.

Over the next four years, she felt she could tell her journal everything. She felt a sense of freedom at being able to do that. For talking was dangerous, didn't Fear tell her that every day? But writing couldn't harm her, could it? Or so she thought.

She was not to blame for the outcome. After all, it was only a small child's naivety that convinced her there was only one key.

Chapter 28

What did I say about Christmas? That there are some words which can trigger my panic attacks. Not only that, but the word 'Christmas' itself does not always conjure up happy memories. Just before the last one, when visitors were due to arrive and were expecting happy faces and an organised house, I had a miscarriage.

All I can remember of it was the searing pain in my womb when I woke up in a small pool of blood. I knew, even before I staggered to the bathroom, what had happened for it had happened before.

Oh, I was not yet so far along the way to having a noticeable bump and attending ultrasounds. I had used one of those home pregnancy tests and grinned with pure happiness when that line went blue; as had my partner, when I told him. We might have our hands full with our two girls, but Patrick and I are young. Even though it wasn't planned, we had welcomed the thought of the new addition tucked away inside me.

Tucked away *safely* was all I hoped for. Don't all expectant mothers wish for that one thing more than anything else? Even though my stomach was flat, it did not stop my hand resting protectively on it. It was in the early hours of that morning when those terrible cramps woke me and I realised that those protective actions had not worked. Even before I climbed out of bed, I already knew – I could feel that emptiness inside me.

It was the third time it had happened. Each loss broke me for a bit, no doubt about it. One second, the baby is in you and you wonder if it's going to be a boy or a girl, perhaps with red hair like Isabelle or dark blonde locks like Sonia. All those questions simply fly into the heads of us expectant mothers, don't they? Will he or she take after me and only eat food when the colours are right and will that tiny person also jump over the cracks in the pavement and hate sand or grass beneath their feet? Those are just some of the questions that I asked myself every day. And it's only by asking myself them that a picture formed in my mind and that blue line on the testing kit I had seen in the bathroom turns into a small person who, within a few months, my partner and I will be meeting. That's the belief which gives me the spirit of happiness I carry around as I picture the child growing inside me.

That was until the cramps and the unwanted flow of blood woke me and I rushed to the toilet. Within seconds, I was looking in dismay at the clots of blood sliding down the inside of the bowl. But then, from the moment I had woken and felt the dampness on my pyjamas, I knew – didn't I? – that he or she was gone and that we would never meet.

That last loss certainly caused my postnatal depression to return. I could hardly bring myself to eat, and tired as

I was, sleep evaded me. In the daytime my greatest wish was to curl up in a ball and just ignore the world. But the world didn't only have me in it, did it? My world also had my partner who shared my sadness and two little girls who needed me. Just thinking of them made my inner voice give me a stern talking-to.

Oh no, you don't, Emily, it said firmly. *Lying in bed wallowing in self-pity is not going to help your children now, is it? They don't deserve a mum who isn't there for them.*

Any loss, especially a miscarriage, can bring on a depression. OK, I accept that, but there's no excuse for not having time for your daughters.

So, no bursting into tears at the slightest thing, they deserve better than that. Remember, they come first, the voice continued. And so it went on, nagging away at me.

Blast, I thought, that inner voice of mine was not going to be quiet until I dragged myself out of bed. Of course I knew it was right, so each morning, I made my legs swing out of that bed, pasted a smile on my sleep-deprived and pinched face, made us all breakfast, before getting out my daughters' toys and books.

I had to make sure that life remained normal for them – they needed me as much as I needed them.

So, feel sad, my voice of Reason told me, *just not in front of them. You didn't have children only to let them down, so get your fighting spirit charged up.*

The one thing my inner voice failed to do was to stop my emptiness allowing another drawer to spring open. One

I have never looked in since I was a teenager. And one most definitely labelled 'Leave Well Alone'.

It was that part of my life that I have tried to erase from my memory. But no matter how hard we try to bury the past, sometimes it refuses to stay forgotten. I remember now that twisting sensation low in my stomach when I heard Carl telling us of his decision that changed so much. Not just for me, but for my mother as well. Up until then, no one could have imagined how he would achieve the results he had aimed for since first meeting us. But then I could not see into his mind and therefore was unaware of just how clearly he could see into mine.

Chapter 29

It was some time before my mother had agreed to marry Carl, not that I think she needed much persuading, when Lily announced to us that she was pregnant. Or rather, it was my dad who told Mum that bit of good news. Knowing who it was on the phone, I had moved close to her, thinking that maybe he wanted to speak to me about that weekend's arrangements. *Fat chance after he shared that particular piece of information!* What was he thinking? I mean, he knew my mother, didn't he? Surely he wasn't expecting congratulations to come down the line, he really should have known there was no chance of that. She just about spat with rage before slamming down the phone the moment the word 'pregnant' penetrated her brain.

'Looks like the slut will be giving you a little brother or sister soon!' she seethed. 'Or did you already know and not tell me?'

'No, Mum. He never said a thing, honestly.'

'Hmm . . . Well, I suppose I'll have to believe you. Anyhow, it's hardly good news for you, is it? I expect your days out with him will come to an end now he'll have another kid to worry about.'

That was my mother, everything always ended up being about her – she just had to get that bit out.

Ignoring the spite in her voice and instead of feeling a baby might be competition, I felt a surge of excitement at the news. At seven, I might not have known much about how babies come into the world, but I did know they were not left behind a bush but grew in their mummy's tummy. Also, it took some time before they arrived. Not that now would have been a good idea to ask Mum how long it would be until I met my new brother or sister. Instead, I kept the smile, which would have shown her just how much I was already looking forward to meeting the new family member, off my face. Once in my room, where I no longer had to listen to her bitching about my dad, my head filled with happy pictures. I saw myself playing with the baby, as I was told my older cousins had done with me, and then when she was a little older, holding her hand to keep her safe as I took her for a walk and reading to her when she was put to bed.

Unfortunately, up to a point, Mum was actually right about me not seeing my dad so much. Not that it was down to him, but Lily – her morning sickness seemed to increase on the weekends I was due to visit. An apologetic phone call would come, telling me not to bring an overnight case as she needed to rest, although most times he also offered to meet me after school on the Friday and take me out for an ice cream.

Being told that I was not going to stay at his house overnight was disappointing. Although I looked forward to seeing him, not to mention loving the large scoops of different flavoured ice cream, the conversation between us was always stilted. I could see him searching hard for something to talk about apart from how was school and what was I learning there.

I too was awkward as I could hardly chat about my mother and Carl. There was too much there I was hiding, and as for the family, because of my stepfather's restrictions on my visits, there was not much I could say to him about them either. And there were times when my conversation also dried up and I too felt uncomfortable. Like Ben, my dad did his best to try to reassure me that he was there for me and I could talk to him about anything if I needed to. But then with Lily using every excuse she could come up with to stop me visiting, it was pretty uncertain as to just what he could do. It was obvious that he would always put her wishes before my needs. All in all, however good the ice cream and cakes in the cafe might be, it was not the best place for us to spend an hour or so.

I can picture him now, light brown hair flopping over his forehead, as with his blue eyes avoiding mine, he glanced discreetly down at his watch before telling me it was time for him to run me home. I think it came as a relief for both of us by then. In contrast, if I was at his house then I spent most of my time upstairs with Lily's son Paul, playing various board games, so he didn't have to think of engaging me in conversation all that much. Surprisingly, Lily didn't seem to mind when the pair of us disappeared up to his room – but then I suppose it gave her more time on her own with her partner.

So yes, she did use morning sickness as a reason to put my visits off. Not that she succeeded every time.

I could see that my father didn't really understand her resentment of me, nor did he face up to the fact that she felt that way. And I know why: it was because I was part of the family he had left for her and she wanted a clean break. Also, I'm sure she never forgot that it was me who caught them in bed together and spilled the beans. I mean, how embarrassing that a four-year-old shows you up? Though I don't think that's an acceptable excuse for a woman who slept with her friend's partner, broke up a family and then was unkind to his seven-year-old daughter. Not that Dad saw any of that, but then we all know that love can be really blind sometimes.

*   *   *

When the day came for Lily to give birth, she was rushed into hospital just in time for an eight-pound baby girl to be delivered.

'Trust her to have such a short labour!' Mum said crossly when she heard. The baby was to be named Crystal, something else Mum was not short on harsh words about. And she made a point of adding the prefix 'half-' to 'sister' whenever the 'Crystal' word cropped up.

I knew about the baby's birth almost straight away. The day after his second daughter arrived in the world, my father came to the school to tell me that I now had a sister. I must say that he was the one person who never prefixed that with the word 'half-' – something that I'm still grateful for, as I was for him coming to the school to tell me about her so quickly. I was so happy, I beamed up at him. He had clearly decided that telling me about her birth over the phone was not the best idea he could come up with. Not after his last experience of speaking to Mum about Lily's pregnancy.

After Dad had told me about Crystal's arrival, I managed to retreat to my room and get out my paints. Only this time I was going to use them for something I wanted to give pleasure. I started making a 'Welcome to the World' card for my sister. Balloons, hearts and a smiley face played a big part in that card. Once finished, and making sure the paint had dried, I hid the card in my satchel. I can just imagine how angry my mother might have been, had she seen it – no doubt she would have snatched it from my hiding place and torn it up.

I actually got a hug from Dad when, on a visit a couple of weeks later, I presented it to him.

'Look, Lily,' he said, showing it to her, 'isn't this thoughtful of Emily?'

'Yes, it's lovely, Emily, thank you,' she said and even managed a tight-lipped smile.

I was, however, far more interested in the tiny bundle lying in Lily's arms than her thanks. Even now I can remember my feelings on seeing that tiny, dark-haired scrap with her tightly closed eyes and rosebud mouth. Just two words came into my head then: 'my sister'.

Oh, how I longed for Lily to ask me to sit next to her so I could hold Crystal just for a few moments!

Not that I dared ask and she didn't suggest it.

The next time I visited, my arms almost stretched out to Crystal of their own volition. Plucking up courage, I did ask if I could sit next to her and just hold her for a moment. Lily's answer, which was repeated often over the next few months, was that her tiny daughter was still too young to be held by anyone who was not an adult.

After the third or fourth time, Crystal's eyes were focusing and her chubby legs were kicking out content-edly. Lily had placed her on the carpet, where she could wave her arms and wriggle away happily. It was when I knelt down beside her that Lily told me sharply to leave her alone. I began to understand the baby's age had lit-tle to do with her refusal to let me hold her – she just didn't want me anywhere near her daughter. This was later confirmed by Paul. With a slight prodding from me, he admitted hearing my dad ask Lily to let me hold the baby, saying that if we were all in the room together, what harm could it do?

'And what did she say to that?' I asked, though I had a pretty good idea.

'Oh, you know Mum!' he told me. 'She glared at him, shook her head and said "No way!" and that was the end of them talking about it.'

* * *

Knowing that Lily was not comfortable with me being in her home saddened me, but I managed to cope with that. Not being allowed to get close to the baby was another matter, though. Lily just did not want Crystal ever bonding with me, that was the nub of the matter. This I knew and not just from Paul. It seems wherever I went, grownups forgot about those sharp little ears of mine. Standing halfway down the stairs, I heard Lily talking to my dad about me. Well, the truth is that I crouched down in an effort to remain invisible as soon as I heard my name mentioned and listened to every word they had to say.

'Look, Ted, I'm just not comfortable with her getting too close to Crystal.'

'Why? We're all in the same room together and it's not as though she's going to drop her or anything.'

'That's not what concerns me. If we let her get too attached now, what are we going to do when they're both a little older? I wouldn't want Crystal picking up any of those peculiar habits of hers.'

'Oh, for heaven's sake, Lily! What habits is a baby going to pick up? She's not exactly talking or doing much now, is she?'

'Look, I know Emily's yours, but you have to admit she's different. And let's face it, as she gets older, she's likely to get even more peculiar. All the fuss with her food and not wanting to walk on different parts of the pavement, that's bad enough, but I've heard her talking to herself as well and you can't say that's normal, now can you?'

'But she's only seven and lots of little kids have imaginary friends, that's something they grow out of.'

'It's not an imaginary friend she's talking to, Ted, she talks to herself! I've heard her telling herself something she has to do. She even tells herself off! That's what doddery old ladies do when they're losing their marbles, not little girls.'

'I just don't see it's a big issue.'

'Well, *I* do! Look, I'm happy enough about her visiting. I don't have a problem her playing with Paul now, do I? He's got used to her odd ways. So, I'm not trying to keep them apart, I just want to monitor it.'

OK, she got most of that right. Not that I considered it was talking to myself when Fear and Reason had an argument and I had to chip in. All right, maybe that is a bit unusual, but it was hardly going to harm a baby, was it? I told myself mutinously, staying very still and listening to what else they had to say.

'The other kids at her school talk about her, you know. Paul's told me that. It's only because her cousins stick up for her that she's not bullied. And that's not what I want for our little Crystal. Children have a knack of copying the older ones. Now, do you see what I mean?'

I heard my father give a resigned sigh: 'Well, she's still my daughter' was his only response and bang, went my hope that he would deny Lily's accusations or at least try and rid her of her concerns. Though I did not believe she really believed them, I was certain it was just another excuse to break all his ties with Mum and me. But that didn't stop my skin prickling at the very thought of the other children who I had believed liked me whispering behind my back.

Don't cry, Emily, whispered Reason, *she'll say anything to get her own way.*

But I was still a child and children want everyone to like them. I swallowed hard and crept away as silently as I could.

I had hoped he might have said more in my defence.

He didn't.

*   *   *

It was soon after I overheard the conversation between Dad and Lily that I noticed the large photo of me had disappeared. As far as I knew, it was the only one that my father had of me. I can still remember it being taken by my uncle on my fifth birthday. He must have got it framed and given it to him – which meant that my mother's family had still been seeing Dad after he left. Not that I was going to let Lily or Mum know that. He had placed it on the mantelpiece in their home and every time I visited, I noticed it was still there – but not any longer. In its place was a professional portrait of Lily, wearing a square-necked white dress and holding a pale pink-clad Crystal.

She must have made him remove it after that last conversation I had managed to overhear.

'Where's my picture?' I asked my dad, looking up at him. He flushed before saying that Lily must have put it away when she was dusting.

A pathetic excuse if ever I heard one, seeing there was another picture in its place.

We both knew that she had done it deliberately.

I had always been aware that Lily had very little time for me but I hadn't realised, despite what she said to my father, how much she disliked having me in her home. Some of it, I was pretty sure, was because my marks at school were always so high, they were remarked on by the teachers. I had seen the expression on her face when my father talked about my achievements with pride and then her getting cross with Paul when he moaned that I was top in everything.

By then I hardly knew what was worse: being unwanted in my father's home or quaking with fear as I tiptoed around Carl in mine.

Chapter 30

I had just turned eight when my mother told me that she was pregnant. She was, I could see straight away, simply overjoyed at the thought and so was I. Whether it turned out to be a brother or a sister, I didn't mind. I knew with a wave of excitement that I would not be separated from paying any attention to this new arrival. He or she would be in our home and there would be no stopping me seeing my sibling every day.

'Are you happy for me, Emily?' she asked and my answer was a wide grin and several enthusiastic nods.

Happy for her? Oh, I was simply overjoyed for both of us – I so wanted a little brother or sister!

For the first time in a long while our smiles were shared. I had never seen her look so happy, not even on her wedding day.

It was after she told me this news that my mum and I became almost close. If I have any good memories of my childhood after Carl came into our lives, it was during those months leading up to my sister's arrival in the world.

After her first scan, Mum brought home a funny-looking picture of something that looked to my eyes like a tadpole.

Of course, to her it looked like her precious baby, who she could hardly wait to meet. She pointed out where the head, arms and feet were, before telling me that the little tadpole was a girl.

'Another daughter,' she said proudly, 'and we're going to call her Maria.'

I felt totally thrilled that I was going to have a sister, a little person I could love and who would love me back.

If my mother was glowing with happiness then I was simply over the moon. For the first time since my dad left, I felt included in her life. Especially as she was happy to chat to me about the baby's progress. I almost danced around the flat with joy after she had shared that news with me. For once nothing I did seemed to annoy her. I have to say too that Carl seemed a different man. Not only was he even more attentive to Mum, but he seemed almost placid. No more outbursts of temper and for the next few months, there was peace and tranquillity in the house.

Or more to the point, he did not hit my mother, or throw her against a wall or place his hands tightly around her neck. He even left me alone, most of the time. There were some evenings when she was resting when he demanded we shower together and I had to put up with him rubbing the whole of my body down and not always through the towel either. Slaps on the legs to remind me just who was in charge of the household continued, but at least that temper of his seemed to be under control.

*   *   *

One of my favourite memories is an evening when Carl was out and my mother let me feel the baby move: 'Come here, love,' she said with a smile and hardly believing my ears, I scuttled over to sit beside her on the settee. 'She's kicking away all right, my active little girl! Here, give me your hand and you can feel her for yourself,' and taking my hand firmly in hers, she placed it on her stomach. At that moment, as we both felt those tiny ripples of movement under our hands, I saw my mother was incandescent with joy and excitement.

'Can you feel her?' she asked.

'Yes,' I whispered, almost dizzy as goose bumps raised up on my arms.

The magical spell was broken when I heard the door open and Carl's voice booming out, though not even he could spoil how I felt.

That night, I went to bed, rolling her name over in my mind, and as I fell asleep, my last thought was how much I was looking forward to meeting Maria.

Chapter 31

I assumed that because Carl and my mother were just so happy about the baby, they would both be pleased that I was as well.

That'll teach me to make assumptions.

There was no way my stepfather, as he insisted referring to himself as, wanted Mum and I to become so friendly. She might not have seen the scowl on his face when he walked in and saw us sitting together, before he quickly replaced it with a smile, but I had. I had seen how he paused just for a moment when he saw our joined hands resting on her stomach. That initial expression gave away his anger at seeing us sitting so close together. I heard Fear muttering, *Look out, he's going to lose it!*

The one thing that must have stopped him finding something to explode about was that he didn't want to upset Mum during her pregnancy. After all, she was in her thirties then, which meant she was not considered a young mother and that in itself could cause complications, so raised fists and loud shouts were out of the question even for Carl. Knowing that the circumstances made his rage impotent gave me a feeling of triumph, although I was careful not to let that show on my face. Mind you, I should have worked out that him having to control his temper was only a temporary occurrence. But then my head was just full of meeting Maria, not worrying about him – another one of my really big mistakes.

'Your mum says you can't wait to meet your new little sister,' he said in the morning when I was getting my breakfast of cereal and juice. 'So, is that right? *Are* you looking forward to having a baby in our home?'

'Oh, yes!' I said, beaming up at him.

I thought he would have been pleased at my response but the mocking smile he gave me in return made my stomach clench as I realised he clearly wasn't.

'Wonderful, isn't it, that your mother's carrying my child! I don't expect you thought that would happen, did you?'

Another of his rhetoric questions where he had no interest in the answer, just giving me his cold fish stare every time he repeated that question, which he did at every opportunity.

'Well, not quite so soon,' was the answer that I could have given, but didn't. After all, only a few weeks had gone by since the wedding, when Mum confided in me that she was pregnant. I sensed, after the scan when I was told it was a girl, that he was still annoyed. All the glee and pride he felt about becoming a father failed to stop him taunting me.

'So, now you will soon have *two* baby sisters to play with, won't you?' he said mockingly when it was the weekend I was to visit Dad.

I hadn't told them about Lily not wanting me to hold Crystal but somehow it seemed he knew. Maybe because I didn't talk about her. When I refused to take the bait, smiled and replied yes, a flash of annoyance flickered across his face.

A small victory, I knew, but I was learning to enjoy them.

'Just remember, if it hadn't been for that court case to get him to support you, you wouldn't be seeing your dad or his family.'

It seemed nothing made my stepfather happier than repeating such unpleasant statements. I could see the enjoyment in his eyes when I flinched. Unfortunately for me, he succeeded with that next accusation in placing a question in my mind – a question that I could not get rid of. Once he had made sure that comment had sunk in, he would give me what he considered was a warm, friendly smile.

'Remember, we are the ones who care for you, Emily. We buy your clothes and feed you – he doesn't. And since your father has obeyed the Court and come back into your life, has he ever bought you anything?'

I thought it better not to mention the ice cream and cakes, so I just shook my head.

'Thought not,' he said triumphantly and that smug smile of his told me he was pleased he had caused me some emotional discomfort.

Not that he was about to let it go at that – he must have really wanted me to feel unloved all right.

'You know, he wasn't just told he had to spend time with you at the court case, don't you? There were other conditions too. Do you know what they are?'

No, I didn't and of course he knew it. With a sinking feeling, I wondered what he was going to say next.

'I'll tell you then,' he continued. 'He was told that as you are his daughter, he has to help provide for you, pay money into your mother's bank account every week. Not that we wanted it for ourselves, I don't want you to think that. You know I look upon you as my daughter, don't you?'

I knew no such thing, which did not stop me nodding my head in agreement instead of speaking.

Nodding was not exactly the same as telling a lie, was it?

'Our plan,' he told me, 'was to put it into a savings account for you. Set you up when you get to school-leaving age. We wanted you to have enough money to buy yourself a nice little flat, that was our plan. Only one thing missing for us to go ahead with that. Guess what it is?'

I just looked helplessly at him, knowing by his smug tone what was coming.

'His payments, that's what. Shows what he thinks of you, doesn't it?'

I wanted to put my hands over my ears and block his voice out, but he would only have caught hold of them and pulled them down. No, it was better to try and stop them entering my mind. I didn't want to believe what he was saying, but then why would he lie? Hadn't he told me so many times that lying was a sin? The adult me now realises that he didn't want me to trust anyone enough to confide in them, but that didn't stop the child me wondering about it for a long time.

Many years later I found out the truth before I went to uni. I finally plucked up enough courage to ask Dad about it and saw the look of anger combined with grief when I told him what Carl had said.

'*What?!* You believed that for all these years?' he said sadly.

Before my dad even showed me the receipts of all the payments he had made during that time, I knew Carl had lied. I think I had known all along, but still there was always that niggling doubt.

'That paid for all your clothes and any presents they gave you, I suppose,' he told me. And I felt his sadness at the huge rift between us that my stepfather had orchestrated.

On the other hand, maybe there were other reasons I was never quite sure if I believed Carl or not. There was no doubt that until I was a teenager, Lily just wished I would disappear into thin air. She had started complaining about the bedroom I slept in as soon as Crystal was born.

'It's all right, her having that room while Crystal is still a baby,' I heard her saying to Dad. 'But what about in a few months' time? She can't sleep in our room for ever, so she will need a room for herself, won't she?'

'Leave it, will you, Lily! Let's wait until she does, shall we?' my father said tiredly, before he did what he had always done when my mother nagged him – picked up his newspaper and buried his head in it. The glare she gave him was almost strong enough to scorch the pages.

Of course, what I had really wanted to hear him say was how important I was to him; that the room would be big enough for two children to share and she should stop making a fuss. Just some words to that effect might have reassured me. But the end result was that she got her way and I was relegated to a folding bed in the dining room – just another sign that made me feel unwanted and that fertilised the doubts Carl had planted.

I wonder if he thought, as I did, that she should have been grateful to me? After all, if I had not spilt the beans, she would not be living with the man she had chased after for so long. Not to mention this time she had produced a baby where the father's name was on the birth certificate. I remember how upset her son Paul was when he found his birth certificate and saw that 'father unknown' was where the father's name should have been.

'I can't believe she didn't know his name, can you?' he had asked me, his face pale with shock.

The answer to that was probably yes. Though what I said instead was maybe he had asked her not to put his name on the certificate. I had learnt that sometimes little white lies are permissible, especially if they are told to protect someone's feelings.

Whatever I thought Lily should have felt, there was no doubt that gratitude did not play any part in it. She complained about my not liking certain colours of food on my plate and repeatedly asked why I could not just eat like everyone else – her son had to, didn't he? But then she said, without caring that I was within earshot, that she was not the only one who thought I was odd and that I made them all feel uncomfortable.

To be fair, my dad did try a couple of times to say that my eating quirks were hardly a problem.

'So, it's OK for you to say that, you're not the one who does the cooking, are you?'

There was no answer to that, just an awkward silence at the table that prevailed while we finished our meal.

Although Lily and I barely tolerated each other, I still wanted to escape my home and spend weekends there. After all, most of the time Paul and I were upstairs playing board games in his room. Looking back, I can see how even before the baby was born, Lily had little time for him. When I scroll through the years to a time I have tried to remove from my memories, I can still see my stepbrother Paul so clearly – a gangly, dark-haired boy with bony knees and elbows, an earnest freckled face and a smile that made his dark green eyes crinkle. Such an empathetic little boy! He understood how I felt about Lily's lack of affection for me and did his best to distract me from it by telling a funny story, or daring me to beat him at a new board game. I think now, with Lily giving so much attention to her new daughter, he might have felt as I did: unwanted and lonely.

As I was not allowed to bring home any school friends – *'They should be doing their homework and not stop you doing yours'* – I was grateful to have Paul as a friend. Common sense told me not to talk too much about him at home though. When his name was mentioned by Carl or my mother, I just shrugged and said, 'He's all right, I suppose.'

Before Crystal arrived, I was so looking forward to having a new sibling. Then once she did, Lily shattered those little girl dreams of mine.

Did my father not know how upset I was when I was never allowed to hold her?

Would I even be allowed to play with her when she was older?

It's not a question I asked him when I was leaving, but it all added up to the reason I did not entirely disbelieve Carl.

Chapter 32

When my mother's bulge was so large that she found it uncomfortable sitting, she tried lying down on the settee. Dark rings circled her eyes, due, she told me, to lack of sleep – 'Your sister just won't stay still, she must be getting impatient to meet us,' she said with a laugh. 'I'm no sooner dozing off than she gives me a kick to let me know she's still awake.'

It was around that time that Gran, knowing Mum was tired, began turning up at weekends with homemade cakes and casseroles. Often my aunts came as well, something that I knew annoyed Carl immensely, as did seeing all the gifts the family kept sending. Little pink outfits and lacy booties seemed to be everywhere. Often, because Mum was working, Gran would meet me at the school gates and walk home with me. Although I still missed going to her house after school, our time together on the journey home did make up for it a little.

* * *

During those last few weeks, my stepdad's chest was puffed up with pride as he bounced around with more energy than

I had ever seen before. Impregnating Mum must have made him feel like a real man. Not only did he escort her when she went for her scans, he even went with her to all those prenatal classes as well.

I just can't imagine him joining in those classes though. You know, the ones where loving partners sit behind, their arms holding bulky bodies? The ones where women are shown the correct way to breathe and their partners encourage them – yes, those classes.

Let's just say I seriously doubted it.

*   *   *

It was just over a week before the due date. My mother and I were ticking off the days on the calendar, both of us excited about meeting the new arrival.

To my delight, it was arranged for me to stay at my grandmother's during the week before the baby was due. I'm sure, had there been another choice, Carl would have taken it. But if my mother had to be rushed into hospital even he could not leave me in the house alone for an indefinite period. Or rather, he would not want the family to know he had. Not when Gran had made her offer of me staying with her until Mum brought baby Maria home. However much I was looking forward to meeting my sister, I relished the thought of having that time with my family.

It was Carl who drove me over on the Saturday.

'Might as well get you settled in,' was all he said to me when he placed my suitcase in the car.

My mother was resting, but nervous at him not being home was the excuse he gave Gran for not stopping, though a charming smile was flashed as he told her how much he and Betty appreciated her help – 'Don't know what we would have done without you,' he added.

Not exactly the sentiment I had heard him express after her visits.

Before he turned around and made his fast exit, he handed over my case and a bag of what he said would be some useful extras for the house. Bending down, he gave me a kiss on the cheek, brushed his fingers lightly on my cheek so I could feel each of those rings against my skin and whispered to me to be good. Then using the cringy 'sweetie' word, he straightened up, patted me on the head and walked to his car.

Lunch with the family followed, as did kicking a ball around with my cousin Ben and being made a fuss of by everyone. No one commented on my eating, or my twisting my hair round my fingers – or anything else for that matter. Instead, they just let me know how happy they were to have me there with them.

Questions were asked about whether I was looking forward to meeting my sister but very little was said about either my mother or Carl, though funnily enough, my father's name came up more than once.

'Are you enjoying spending time with him?' I was asked. I told them I was and then filled them in about him often taking me out for cakes and ice cream. When I told them that, I noticed them glancing at each other. I think they'd worked out this was not something Carl or my mother ever did with me. As I seldom did anything interesting on those weekends when they made an excuse not to join the family, I was relieved they did not ask me about them – I guess they all knew it was just that Carl didn't want to come.

I'm sure too they could all see just how happy and relaxed I was to be with them. Some of my old confidence had returned and without being aware of Carl watching my every move, I found myself chatting away non-stop. Also, I wasn't dreading the phone ringing to summon me home. I was where I was happy to be and not just for a couple of hours either, but a whole week or even longer.

In my gran's house nothing had changed. There was no one telling me to do my homework or saying that television was bad for me. Later, when bedtime came, I was allowed to read a little by the reading lamp that Gran left on for me. Feeling safe and cared for, I finally drifted off to sleep with a smile on my face as I thought about the sister I would soon be meeting.

Chapter 33

All that week of being with Gran, I felt so spoilt – there was homemade cake when I came back from school, my favourite meals were cooked for supper and the television was turned on for us both to watch.

It was she who told me after I had been there a few days that my mother had been taken to the hospital and given birth to her daughter.

'When are they coming home?' I asked.

'Not for a few days, dear. Your mum needs some more rest.'

'And then she will bring Maria home with her?'

'Maria might have to stay a little longer,' Gran told me gently.

'Why?'

'Oh, just to make sure she's strong and healthy.'

'Is there something wrong with her?'

It was not often my gran was at a loss for words, but she was this time. I just knew she was holding something back. Aunt Lizzy came and stayed one evening when Gran went to visit my mother, but as I had not heard her come home, she must have stayed a long time.

Which wasn't usual, was it?

Understanding that I was unlikely to stop bombarding her with questions if she didn't tell me more, she sighed a little and explained that Maria was slightly delicate: 'She just needs to get a bit stronger before she can leave hospital,' she said in an attempt to be reassuring.

Now, eight-year-olds might not be unduly sensitive, but they can spot an evasion when they hear one. So, I was not as satisfied with her answer as she might have wished, although common sense told me that I was not going to get any more information from her.

Later the same day, Carl turned up. If I hadn't realised just how ill my baby sister was, his appearance told me everything. The grey-faced man who came into Gran's sitting room was not the Carl I had ever seen before. For the first time since I had met him, with his creased shirt and dark stubble on his chin, he looked almost dishevelled. All the bounce had left him and instead of his overly confident self, he looked both tired and worried.

I wondered why he had come because I would hardly be going back with him if Mum was still in the hospital. He didn't offer any explanation for his visit, just slumped on the settee and gratefully took the cup of tea Gran had quickly made.

'Betty is staying in for a few days longer,' he told her. 'She just doesn't want to come home without the baby.' And did I really see the moisture in his eyes as he said that? I think I did.

Just when I was wondering again why Mum would be told to go home without the baby, he asked my grandmother if I could stay a little longer, explaining, 'I need to be at the hospital with Betty as much as possible.'

Gran said of course I could and I tried not to look too pleased that I did not have to leave yet. At eight, I just did not understand that Maria, who had been born after the full nine months, was likely to be very ill if she had to be kept in the hospital. But then, I had no way of knowing that the moment she entered the world, her blue-tinged face rang every alarm bell in the delivery room. She was whisked away to the neonatal clinic so quickly, she hardly had time to utter her first cry.

Today, I can picture my mother, arms aching to hold her daughter, being told the reason why her baby was not with her. Even now, after all she did to me, I can still feel some pity. As a little girl, I was unaware of what was happening though. There was only so much information my gran thought should come my way. I had not been told that the baby was on a ventilator while the surgeons discussed the nature of the operation she needed on her heart with her distraught parents. If anything, I was upset that I had not been taken to see her – I knew my grandmother and my aunts were visiting, so why couldn't I go too?

Even if they had told me more, I would not have understood what Mum was going through though. How when she went to her daughter's cot, she had to look at all those tubes inserted into that tiny frame. She must have longed to be able to hold her, but Maria was just too fragile and the only part of her she could hold was her hand. It was not surprising that she barely rested during the weeks Maria was in there – if it had been my child, I would hardly have left her side either.

Of course, my eight-year-old self was repeating the same questions excitedly to her grandmother.

When can I see her? What does she look like and when is she coming home?

My very patient gran kept telling me that she was still poorly and I could visit her when she was a little better. What she did not tell me about was the heart condition that Maria had been born with.

After another week had gone by, Mum came home from the hospital and for the next three weeks, I went to and fro between my home and Gran's. I found it hard to concentrate at school, though I did manage to do my homework.

If Carl had appeared looking tired and dejected when he came to Gran's, my mother seemed even worse. Although it was mid-winter, she was constantly wearing sunglasses. This was very strange to me. I only realised later on that it was to hide her swollen eyes. She was smoking a lot too, which was not something that she normally did. I heard them reassuring each other, saying the doctors were doing everything they could. Mum was trying to convince both Carl and herself as well that the doctors would save her. For those three weeks she lived in hope – or rather, perhaps I should say, she *tried* to.

It seemed her time was split between telling whichever one of us was in earshot that everything was going to be all right and that soon, she would be bringing Maria home to either bursting into tears or, with shaking hands, lighting up a cigarette. During that time, I hardly saw her without a cigarette or a sodden tissue in her hand. Although most of the time was spent at the hospital, she did try and rest when she drifted back into the home. It was then I would hear her sobbing and sobbing; that sound made me start to cry as well.

It was then that my gran told Carl very firmly that she wanted to take me to the hospital to see Maria.

'Why, exactly?' he asked in a disinterested tone.

'Because, Carl, Maria is Emily's sister and she should see her.'

'*Half*-sister, you mean. But take her if you must.'

Placing a hand on his arm, Gran just said, 'Thank you, Carl.'

He must have known then the reason she insisted I went with her. Gran had already told me that Maria was in a Special Unit and that she was still very ill. On the way to visit her, she also explained about the ventilator and what it was for. She tried her best to prepare me for what I was going to see when I got there – the tubes that were helping my sister breathe and receive food and other liquids containing medicine that were there to make her better.

Gran had explained that I would have to look through a glass panel but nothing she told me could ever really prepare me for the sight of my new baby sister. Tubes seemed to be attached to every part of her tiny, unmoving frame.

Tears spurted from my eyes as I gazed at her.

'They are trying to make her better, Emily,' Gran told me as she placed an arm around my shoulders.

But they didn't.

She was just under a month old when she died.

It was my mother who told me. Not face-to-face, so I could offer her some comfort. Instead, she chose to do it by phone. In a cold dispassionate voice that was almost a whisper, she told me, 'Maria died during the night.'

I have only a blurred memory of what happened after that – I can't remember when I went home or who took me there. Just that not long after that call, I was back.

* * *

I did ask myself why my mum and Carl had not left me with my gran – they certainly did not seem to welcome my presence. Since Mum had come home from hospital it was as though in all her efforts to save my sister, she had completely forgotten my existence.

Over the remaining years I lived with her, it was as if I was a mere memory of a past life, one that didn't matter anymore – I was there, but somehow invisible to her. While she had been spending time with Maria, I had been an inconvenience to her busy hospital life. Even when she was in our home with me, her mind was exclusively with my sister.

She only seemed to know how to be a mother for Maria.

After Maria's death, it seemed that neither Mum nor Carl could look at me. Now I can understand my mother's grief and accept that my stepfather was also devastated – after all, even monsters have feelings, but then their grief unsettled me. Children do not see adults as people who can break down without warning, they think they are invincible. It would never enter a young child's head that sometimes adults too can be incapable of handling what life throws at them. So, if I didn't fully understand what they were going through, neither did they recognise my grief.

So, yes, I do empathise with the pain my mother must have felt after losing her child – I cannot imagine anything more horrific for a woman to endure. As I have said earlier, I have gone through three miscarriages myself and that is nothing close to losing the child you have given birth to. It would break the strongest person, and it broke her.

Chapter 34

Dear Diary
    So very sad because Maria is dead. We all are and it's horrid in the house. I think Mum wishes it was me who had died, not Maria. I think he does too. Then he would have a perfect little girl instead of me, who is not one.

*   *   *

I can't remember how many days it was before the funeral when Carl came home from visiting Mum's family just about shaking with rage. I think it was no more than a couple of days, but so much of that time is a blur and memories do get jumbled.

He had left saying he just wanted to go over a few details with them about the funeral. My mother didn't ask what details he was referring to, or suggest that he could pick up the phone instead of driving over. Since Maria had died she was, for the most part, too wiped out on medication to question him.

After he left, she hardly uttered a word. Not that this was too unusual. Most of the time she was either in her bedroom with the curtains closed and the lights off, or sitting staring unblinkingly into space. I too sat silently, listening to the eerie silence in the flat. Mum had no interest in switching on the television or tuning in the radio to one of the music stations she loved. I had tried to talk to her, but even when I asked a simple question, such as could I get her anything or make her a cup of tea, I seldom received an answer. She did not even turn her head when I entered the room. Mealtimes were completely dismal too – she picked at her food or pushed it to one side. If her sisters or Gran hadn't brought over their casseroles and home-baked pies, I don't know what we would have eaten.

Carl, too, hardly said a word, apart from telling me to remove the dishes from the table or clean something, and in the end, I couldn't find any words to break the silence. Their grief weighed too heavily in the air, the weight of it pressing down on me every waking hour. My sleep was interrupted by dreams, and during the daytime I felt both disconsolate and listless.

In my room, using my new silver pen, I had begun to write down my feelings in my diary. It had become my friend, the one I could share everything with. When I look back on those entries, I can see the start of my younger self's depression. Now I call it the 'Black Dog', one that can sneak up and nip at our heels and the same one famously suffered by Winston Churchill. But dogs can be trained to stop their misbehaviour, can't they? They just need a firm hand. It was only when I learnt to look forward and not behind me that I finally mastered how to make it obey me.

I remember my schoolwork suffered. I could not concentrate, words blurred in front of my eyes and made no sense, and the answers to those Maths questions suddenly refused to jump into my head. The teachers were very understanding, but it still bothered me that I was not getting the marks I was used to. The Head sat me down in the privacy of her office and asked if I wanted to talk about how I felt about my sister's death. She gently explained that it was natural to grieve. And although I just nodded instead of opening up, she reassured me that if I needed to talk at any time, her door was always open.

But it was a door that I never did walk through voluntarily.

* * *

I knew from Ben that our grandmother had asked Carl to let me go and stay with her. She had told him that I was too young to cope with their grief as well as mine and that I would be better off spending some time with my cousins, who would try and cheer me up over the weekend.

'And what did he say?' I asked when Ben told me all this.

'What do you think? Of course, he said no, that your place was with them and they both understood that you needed attention and so on and so on. Gran also said she was worried about your mum, that she had seen she was not coping at all. She mentioned a grief counsellor – you know, that's someone you can talk to if you are unhappy. He just laughed at that. Said she had pills from the doctor which were doing the trick and she had her mother and her sisters to talk to.'

'How do you know all that?'

'How do you think? My mum told my dad when we were having supper. Anyhow, how is your mum really?'

'Bad, Ben, really bad,' I said sadly. 'She cries a lot. I was told to pack away all of the new little baby outfits people had sent over so she wouldn't have to see them. And then she wanted to know where they were, told me to bring them to her and she just sat there stroking them and crying.'

'Sounds just awful, especially for you.'

'It is.'

Chapter 35

Over the coming months, the belief that my mother felt the wrong daughter had died steadily grew in my head, so it's little wonder that this was one of the saddest times in my life. During her pregnancy, I had felt a closeness growing between us, only for it to disappear instantly. I had spent weeks imagining having a baby sister and stood in the hospital with a lump in my throat when I saw her. From that one time I felt such a surge of love that I prayed every night that the doctors would make her better. Not that I really believed in God – my gran had never managed to persuade me that He heard our prayers. But after Maria's death, any scrap of faith I had in the man who lived above the clouds withered and died.

The night when Carl came back from visiting Mum's family, I still believed that our lives could not get any worse. *Wrong again.* By the end of that evening, I had found out it could. It started with the sound of the front door slamming so loud, it made me jump. Even before he called out, the noise alone warned me that all was not well. A sense of dread made me sit bolt upright, hands under my knees as in those loud, aggressive tones of his he called out for my mother.

My stomach twisted with apprehension as Fear muttered, *Yup, there's trouble coming.* For using that tone of voice was something Carl did when his mood was darker than a night's starless sky. As the flat was scarcely large, it was hardly something he needed to do. He did it solely to make us quake in fearful anticipation before he told us what the problem was.

Before I could try and guess just what had angered him to such an extent, I heard him yell, 'Emily, get in here now!' My legs shook when I stood and left my room. *Surely there was nothing wrong I had done?* A thought that wouldn't prevent an icy chill touching my neck as reluctantly, I walked into the sitting room.

As soon as I entered, I could see how flushed Carl's face was and how those cold grey eyes glittered with rage. Whatever he had managed to say to my mother before he shouted out my name seemed to have had very little impact on her. She was staring up at him almost blankly. Not much of what went on around her penetrated her pill-taking haze – something else that increased his temper.

'Emily, get your mother some strong coffee. She needs to be able to listen to what I've got to say and so do you,' he instructed.

Thanking my lucky stars that his anger had little to do with me, I sped into the kitchen and returned with a cup of steaming coffee that I handed to Mum. Carl barely took his eyes off her as she very slowly sipped it. I began to wonder if she was using a delaying tactic to put off hearing the tirade that he was waiting impatiently to release. Clearly, he wanted us to recognise that he was furious about something or someone. In no time at all, he would be pouring out details of his dislike for whoever had upset him in the time he had been out. Yet there was a difference in the anger he was showing that night, something in it that did not quite ring true. Even at eight, I was able to question the performance unfurling before me.

'Are you fully awake now, Betty?' he snapped when her last drop of coffee had finally been swallowed.

'Yes, Carl.'

'Good,' he said and then stood in between us and almost shouted out the string of venomous words that caused my mother to lose even more colour from her cheeks and me to start trembling throughout my body. Not that I can remember every single word, but much as I would like to wipe his words from my mind, I can remember the gist of them all right.

Having both an echoic memory, which means I can remember conversations word-for-word, as well as a photographic one, is not always as useful as we think!

'They all refused to lend us a single penny to help with the funeral,' were the first words he spat out.

Mum suddenly woke from her daze. She might not love me, but I knew her sisters and her mother were important to her and who else could he be referring to?

'What are you saying, Carl? That you went to my family for help and they refused you? I can't believe that! For heaven's sake, they have all been really supportive – looked after Emily, brought round meals for us and Mum was a brick when I was spending all that time in hospital. There must be some mistake. Let me ring Lizzy, she'll know what's going on.'

Using her hand to push herself up, she moved towards the phone, though not fast enough for him. He spun round and stood in front of her, his bulk preventing her from moving any closer.

'Oh no, you don't, Betty! You just do what you do best, sit there, do nothing and listen to me,' he instructed her.

I saw her recoil at the sudden savage expression on his face.

'Your family, I'm telling you now, they are no longer ours. Do you get it? What exactly have they ever done for us anyhow? And don't say looking after that daughter of yours. They spoil her rotten so she gives me even more work to do. They refuse to accept she's a complete retard and an embarrassment to you. She needs to do homework, but no, they let her watch those stupid television programmes instead. Well, no more of that! She's old enough now to get herself back from school.

'Do you hear me, Emily?' he said, turning to me. 'No more visiting that grandmother of yours.'

But I could only stare at him. Nothing he was saying made sense – apart from what he really thought of me, that was. Hearing that part of the conversation, I felt as though a hole had been dug under my feet. I crossed my arms, pushed my right hand under my upper left arm and pinched the soft flesh as hard as I could.

Feeling pain was preferable to crying.

Not that Mum looked outraged by his opinion of me, it was the disagreement with her family that gave her concern.

'You're going to have to decide, Betty, it's them or me.'

'But, Carl . . .'

'No buts, they insulted me.'

'Carl, I don't know what happened. I wasn't there, was I? I don't even know who it was you were talking to.'

'It was both your brother-in-laws. Your brother didn't even bother to come to the house although I had asked him to. After all he said at our wedding, just puff! He sent a message saying he can't help. I had explained earlier that I had a bit of a cash flow problem and asked if they could help, just to tide us over, so they knew exactly what I was coming for. They had told me they would have to talk it over with their wives first, your lovely sisters. So, when I went over, it was to go over the costs.

'I've never asked them for help before. And if it was just for me, I wouldn't have. But this was just as much for you. And our daughter, our little Maria.'

The moment her name left his lips he looked down, his shoulders shook and pulling a hanky out of his pocket, he hastily blew his nose very hard.

'I'm sorry,' he added, 'it's just that even speaking her name chokes me up. I know I should have asked you to ask them, but I didn't think you were strong enough.'

'But you never told me there was a problem with money.'

'No, well, I didn't want to worry you at the moment. It's just a bit of a cash flow problem, that's all. I explained all that to them. There will be money in the coffers again next month.'

'OK, Carl, but what exactly did they say? There must have been more to it than you're telling me,' she persisted.

'If you must know, though I didn't want to tell you, they said that they had helped you enough when you split up with Ted. This time they were not going to put their hands in their pockets, we would have to sort everything out ourselves. Anyhow, now you have it, that's what they said.'

I just wished I could go to my room, anything to get away from them. Surely none of this was anything to do with me?

'Now, Betty, are you still saying you don't believe me?' he went on.

'No, of course not, Carl, but I still don't understand it.'

'Well, I know they've never liked me, but I never thought they wouldn't do it for you. I knew they always wanted to see us split up. They don't think I'm a good enough stepfather for that stupid girl of yours, think I'm too strict with her.'

'Who said that?'

'Your mother, who else? But if it had been that girl needing money,' he said, nodding scornfully in my direction, 'trust me, their hands would have gone in their pockets all right! But then, she's not my daughter, is she? So, don't you go thinking that if you make that phone call, they will open up their cheque books. You'll just be humiliated like I was.'

I could see the tears running down my mother's face at what he was saying. Every word was wounding her to the core. She must have been desperate to pick up the phone and talk to either of her sisters or her mother – there was no doubt they were important to her, something that Carl had resented ever since he came into our lives. As for me, I was just thankful that he had only used words as weapons when he had hurled that barrage of them in my direction. If he had asked me one question, I could not have uttered a word – I just felt numb. Not all of it had sunk in, but it would later on.

'Carl, please let me speak to Mum at least,' my mother said pleadingly. 'I can't believe that she wouldn't help us!'

'No need for you to call her and beg, Betty. I've already got the money,' he said with what I detected to be a note of smugness. 'Went to a friend of mine, a proper friend, who gave it to me straight away. And you know the only question he asked me? Was it enough?'

Carl had watched any last semblance of defiance in my mother dwindle away and now he announced his rules for how we were to act towards everyone in her family.

As soon as the funeral was over, they were to be cut from our lives completely.

'So, you can go and visit if you like, Betty, but what would that tell me? That you're not on my side, that's what! For your sake, I will have to put up with them being there when we bury our daughter. If it had been up to me, I would have told them all not to come. As far as I'm concerned, they're not welcome. But I understand that would cause you more distress.

'If you want to pick up the phone and have your daily chat, feel free, but just remember what that will tell me – that you don't mind how they spoke to me and how they humiliated me. So, what's it going to be, you're on their side against me?'

Mum tried to protest, not that Carl had any interest in listening to her arguments. Instead, he carried on ranting for at least another hour until she was totally exhausted. In the end she capitulated, murmuring gently, 'Your side, of course.'

One down and one to go was how Carl must have looked at this victory when he finally turned his attention to me.

'As for you, Emily, the same rules apply,' he told me. 'I'll take you to school and you can now bring yourself home. You know the bus route, don't you? So, no more pally-pally with that Ben you like so much. No doubt he or your grandmother will be down that school, looking for you. So, if I hear you've been meeting them, or going to your gran's house, I think you know what punishment you'll be in for. You understand me?'

I did.

'So, now you know what it is I want you to do when either of them turn up?'

The feeling of dread that was beginning to curl around my heart told me the answer he wanted to hear from me, but still, I waited for him to say it.

'You are to walk away, you understand me?'

'Yes,' I whispered.

'That's your mother's wish as well as mine, isn't it, Betty?'

'Yes, Carl,' she said softly, but those two words did not convince me. I could tell by the tears prickling her eyes that she just wished this was not happening.

'Carl,' she said hesitantly, interrupting this tirade, 'how are we to act at the funeral? We'll just have to pretend everything's all right, won't we? It would look really bad if we didn't.'

I held my breath, waiting to see what he would say.

'Yes, all right,' he said reluctantly.

'And you,' he said, turning to me, 'you just keep that mouth of yours shut when you go to school tomorrow, OK? No repeating what you've just heard. I'll find out all right if you have! I'll pick you up from school. Just tomorrow, mind. Don't expect me to do that often.'

I didn't.

That was the end of the conversation.

Carl had finally got what he wanted.

I wonder now just when he had decided to put that plan into action and how he could bring himself to use his own child's death to achieve it. There's no doubt in my mind that he was completely aware of my mother's fragile state and took full advantage of it.

She was simply devastated by the death of Maria. I had seen those damp patches on her blouse that night when he let forth all his venom. Then I didn't know what they were. Now I know that she was still producing milk for a baby who was no longer there, one she had never been able to breastfeed. Carl would have known that too. I imagine she cried every time her breasts leaked the nutrition her baby had never needed. She was simply incapable of making decisions or standing up for her family, me or herself. But that was how Carl's mind worked – no one else in our lives had to matter.

I can remember when Mum and I first moved into what was then our shabby flat. Outside was a small playground with a couple of swings and a climbing frame. She used to let me play there, and before he came I was out there all the time. Mum and I got friendly with one of the neighbours. We both really liked her, but he didn't. He said she was common and that all she did was drink coffee and smoke – '*A bad influence on Emily*' – and he didn't want us mixing with her.

And that was that – we just never saw her anymore.

Nor did I play outside again.

Chapter 36

What do I remember about the funeral? I've been asked. Nothing, I was not there is the short answer. I have no idea what happened when my mother met her family – I guess she was too upset to show anything but grief for the death of her baby. That doesn't mean I don't have clear pictures in my head of some parts of that day. I can still see my eight-year-old self, almost in tears at being excluded from the funeral. She was trying not to protest at Carl and her mother's decision that she was too young to attend a funeral. But still, despite Carl's warning, she managed to blurt out that Gran and the family would expect to see her there.

She knew it was the wrong plea when Carl's eyes darkened.

'And what did we discuss just a couple of nights ago?' At those words, which brought that night sharply back into focus, all she could do was not let those tears out. The dreadful things he had said had kept her awake for most of the night, although the reality hadn't really sunk in yet. She had heard him explode before and then it was all forgotten.

Surely this time would be the same? Not that that made everything he had said to her go away.

I can still see him standing between Mum and me, hurling those wounding words around the room; I could even hear the underlining tinge of triumph in every syllable. Another picture suddenly came into my mind, one that made the hairs on the back of my neck stand up: Carl on his birthday, standing across the lawn from us and staring daggers at Ben and me, and all we were doing was chatting. Both of us had seen the thunderous expression on his face when he thought no one was looking. We had recognised the fact that he disliked seeing us together, but neither of us had thought of what his reason could have been.

Remembering that incident caused a glimmer of suspicion to float into my thoughts, a glimmer that before the day was out had crystallised into a full-blown belief.

Maybe Carl was scared that I would confide in Ben, if I met him at the funeral. He would not have been able to keep me glued to his side all the time, would he?

A couple of his business friends were attending – '*to give me support*'. He had also implied that it was one of those men who he had borrowed the money from, so he would have had to spend some time with them. And he wouldn't have wanted to appear to be acting strangely by insisting I stayed by his side – not with those friends of his there.

I might not have had the vocabulary at that age to put my understanding of his actions into words, but I knew instantly what Carl was really up to: he resented not being the only person of importance in Mum's life. But more than that, he didn't want anyone else to have any influence either. Likewise, he didn't want me to become closer to my cousins, especially one who was several years older.

Just what might I tell him, given the opportunity? And maybe, just maybe, Mum and I would have found out that he had lied.

The next snapshot that comes into my mind of that day of the funeral is Carl and my mother walking into the sitting room, dressed all in black. Not only was Mum wearing a knee-length skirt and a short boxy jacket, she also had a black pillbox hat with a veil that hid her eyes perched on her head. It was new and I suspected her sisters must have taken her out shopping.

Carl had arranged for one of his friends' wives – another blonde in a tight dress and high heels – to sit with me. What was it with these wives? Why was it so hard to tell one from the other? And it was always apparent that they were all a lot younger than their husbands.

'Hello,' she had said, 'I'm Sally. I'm going to keep you company. Anything you would like to do?'

Yes, go to my room and ignore you.

'We could watch television,' I told her as brightly as I could manage, thinking at least I would not have to make any conversation then. To be fair, she did her best. She asked me to choose what I wanted to watch, not that I really had any desire to watch anything – I wanted to be at the funeral where I could say goodbye to my sister.

Sally made me some lunch and tried her best to chat with me. And I, realising the despondent mood I was in was not her fault, made a little effort too and thanked her for making my lunch.

I can remember when they came back, though. Mum was weeping uncontrollably, her whole body shaking with grief. And Carl seemed to be holding her up and with his arm around her, led her to the bedroom. Sally made a hasty exit and that left me alone with him.

He told me that it was Mum's family who had organised all the food and drinks for the mourners. 'That's the last time I will have to talk to them,' he said with that smirk that repulsed me.

I mean, how two-faced was that? Letting them supply all the food and drinks when he was planning to make them all disappear from our lives within a few hours?

'Now, you remember what we discussed the other night, don't you, Emily?'

'Yes.'

Of course, I had hoped that this proclamation was just a show of temper and he would relent, but his next sentence told me there was no chance of that.

'I expect you to obey those rules completely, starting from tomorrow. Have I made that clear enough?'

'Yes.'

'Good.'

And as he said it, he smiled at me – the one that showed his teeth, but never quite reached his eyes.

'I know this has been hard on you, Emily, and very hard on your mother too, but we will get through it, we are still a family.'

I kept my face as blank as I could.

Had he forgotten what he said about me such a short time ago? He might be able to dismiss it, but I couldn't.

And I never did.

I went to my room then. Lay on the bed dry-eyed with my fists clenched hard, wishing the next day would never come.

After some lapse of time, he called out to me, saying he had left some food out and it was on the table – he was just going to see how my mother was. I didn't want any food, but knowing it would infuriate him if I ignored him, I tiptoed out.

So, I ate alone on the day of my sister's funeral. Then I washed my plate and took myself to bed, that I remember. But not as much as I have perfect recall of what came later. I was reading with my bedside light on when I heard his footsteps coming down the hall: he was still awake. Quick as a flash, my light went off, the book I had been staring at disappeared under my pillow and I curled up as tightly as I could.

If he looks in, he will think I'm asleep, I thought to myself.

I heard the click of my bedroom door opening, then I smelt the waft of his aftershave and with a shudder, I knew he was in my room. *Oh, please,* I said to myself silently, *please don't tell me to get out of bed and take a shower with you.* Even at eight, I already knew that taking me into the bathroom had little to do with getting clean. It was all about power, wasn't it? Not that I understood that when I was still that little girl. All I knew was that Fear had also entered the room alongside the man who, with his beatings and threats, was responsible for it seldom leaving me alone.

It was that little demon who made me obey Carl's commands and place a smile of enjoyment on his face when, without a murmur, I obediently followed him into the bathroom. He took great delight in watching me, my face burning with shame, standing naked before him; he enjoyed touching me everywhere, and not always through the towels either. I'd seen that gloating expression on his face when he saw how I tried to avert my eyes from looking at his body with that ugly red thing sticking out, felt his breath quicken against my neck when my body was pressed tightly against him and sensed his approaching excitement as he ground himself harder against me. I just hoped he would believe I was asleep and go away if I lay completely still and tried to breathe deeply.

None of that fooled him.

'I know you're still awake, Emily,' said his voice coming from above my head and I knew my wish had not been granted, he was not going to leave.

'You can't fool me, can you?' his voice told me, and I felt cold air against my back and then the mattress seemed to be sinking as he lifted the duvet and crawled in.

'Thought I would spend some time with you. You've been on your own all day, haven't you?'

I wish.

'Your mother's taken a sleeping pill. She won't wake up until morning and I think we both need some company.'

But it wasn't company he wanted – well, not like a social chat. He wasn't going to ask me what I might want to talk about, was he? He could have asked if I wanted to hear about the funeral, not what they had to eat afterwards. If he had, I could have used my imagination to picture the coffin being lowered into the ground, heard the minister's prayer and watched as my mum threw a soft toy into the grave to keep her company. Then, with that image in my head, I might have said my final farewells. But that was not what he had in mind: he had neither interest nor compassion for my own grieving, the only people who would have understood were the very ones I was now forbidden to talk to.

He's not going away, Fear muttered, *just stay silent*.

So, I did – my body was so stiff that I could not have moved, not even when his hands gripped the backs of my shoulders, drawing me firmly against his own body. I could feel puffs of his warm breath on my cheeks and the smell of his aftershave was stronger. It filled my nose and seemed to enter my throat, making me feel nauseous – it always did, even when I smelt it in a room that he had just left. I tried to hold my breath to stop it.

'Is this what you and Ben get up to when my back is turned?' he asked as his hands fumbled under my pyjamas. 'I think it is and that you enjoy it.'

I wanted to say no, that I didn't know what he was talking about, but Fear kept me silent. That part of him I hated was digging in my back while his hands ran up and down my body and then snaked down lower to touch me between my legs. I wanted to wriggle away but his other arm was holding me so tightly, it was impossible to move. He grunted in my ear and his body shook against mine.

'You'll get to like me being nice to you,' he said, his fingers still stroking my chest.

Please go, was all I could think. *Please, please!*

I finally felt him sitting up, then he was out of my bed.

'Don't forget about tomorrow,' he told me, and then I could hear him fumbling for his clothes until at last, the door clicked behind him.

My hands grasped the pillow and I buried my head in it to choke back the scream shooting up through my body. I just knew that if I opened my mouth and allowed it to escape, it would fill the room with all the anguish trapped inside me.

Dear Diary

He came into my room this time. Said I might need company because I had been on my own all day and gave me a cuddle. That sounds all right, doesn't it? But it's not. Not when he takes his clothes off and gets in beside me.

That thing that boys pee with is forced into my hand. Hot and slimy, it makes me feel sick. He holds my fingers over it, forces my hand up and down until my hands are sticky – sticky with something that comes out of him. It leaves damp patches and clings to my skin.

Ugh, it's so gross! And it smells horrid.

When he left, I had to move away from that damp patch he'd left behind.

Chapter 37

I couldn't bring myself to face Ben and then walk away without saying anything. How could I? He was my closest friend. Out of all my cousins, I felt he really 'got me'. He never once said anything when I avoided white lines. In fact, he laughed, held my hand and helped me jump over those sections on zebra crossings, making it feel that it was a game we were both playing. Nor did he ever tease me about my eating habits or mention my sucking my tongue when stressed, which I was each time he took me home. And if he had heard me talking to myself, which I'm sure he had, he just acted as though it was perfectly normal.

Understanding my confidence needed building, he made a point of telling me his teacher had referred to me as his 'clever little cousin' – 'Oh, come on! You must know you are,' he said, nudging me in the ribs when I looked doubtful. I could hardly bear the thought of not spending any more time with him, he had looked out for me ever since I could remember.

When Ben was given the task of taking me home each night as soon as the phone rang, he would give me that smile that lit up his face and bounce over to where I was sitting: 'Come on, Sprat, journey time,' he would say as he pulled me up. I knew that he was totally aware that I hated that journey home and I really wanted to stay where I was. That's why he tried to turn it into a joke and chatted to me right up until we were outside the door. Then he would give my shoulders a squeeze and say, 'Night, Sprat, see you tomorrow.'

I felt physically sick at the thought of ignoring him. In fact, I knew I wouldn't be able to do it if I saw him. *What? Stick my head in the air and walk away as Carl had told me?* He would just think it was me playing a game and chase after me. And then what would I do? I was not allowed to say that Carl had told me to ignore the family and that if I was being loyal to him, it had to be my decision. If I continued walking away from Ben, I knew he would grab hold of me and demand an explanation – not that he wouldn't immediately guess who the person behind my actions was.

I could just imagine the questions he would fire at me if I tried to get away from him. He had a knack of quizzing me about Carl, or rather 'your mother's new man', as he called him. I had guessed from some of his questions that he had never taken to my stepfather. In fact, I knew he was suspicious of him. He was pretty sure I was not being treated properly and persisted in asking me questions as to how he was towards me. But what could I say without bringing trouble down on my shoulders? So, I kept quiet.

I had learnt from a very young age that loose-lipped mouths cause nothing but problems, hadn't I?

Had Carl not thought that he would be blamed for my actions? No one would think I had thought of it all by myself. But then, that was something for him to work out.

Mine was to avoid punishment.

* * *

I decided that the only way I could avoid Ben was by darting out through the back of the school. There was a pathway there leading to a small padlocked gate. I would have to climb over it, but that would be better than going out through the main gates where my cousin would be waiting. When the final bell rang, I sped as fast as I could to that gate and once over it, ran all the way to the bus stop. Luckily, I was tall for my age so I looked older than eight – children as young as me were seldom unaccompanied on public transport.

How I wished, as I did so often, that I had never walked into my parents' bedroom that day. If I hadn't seen anything or even kept quiet, I wouldn't have to look at the face I disliked so much over the breakfast table every morning. Nor would I be forced to listen to his demands as he announced different ways of taking away my access to the people I loved.

But then no one can undo what's done, can they?

Ben must have realised very quickly how I was managing to avoid him. On the third day, what I was most dreading happened: Gran turned up. Not at the school gates, but by the padlocked one. For a moment I stood stock-still, wondering what to do. I knew she had seen me. No point sprinting back to the main gates either, I was pretty sure that Ben would be waiting there. I felt waves of panic as I realised that I was trapped.

I just knew that if I stopped and talked to her, Carl would find out. I didn't know how he managed it, but he had an uncanny knack of knowing exactly what I did each day. He had already praised me for not talking to Ben – I didn't have a clue how he knew that. I only confided in my diary and that was locked, right?

Now, what did I say about that little demon Fear removing all rational thought? All I had to do was run up to Gran, ask her to let me stay and tell her everything that was happening at home. Within a nanosecond, the family and social workers would have been hammering down Carl's door. In fact, my guess now is that if I had told my gran everything that day, the family and my real dad might just have gone to visit Carl first, before handing him over to the police. Which would hardly have been difficult with having an uncle in the force, would it? But then I didn't know that my stepfather was breaking the law, so rational thought refused to put up a fight, but Fear did. It whispered to me just how bad my punishment would be if I stopped and talked to her.

Just climb over that gate and run, it told me.

And that's exactly what I did.

'Emily,' I heard her say, 'what's the matter, love?' And her hand reached out to me as I climbed down.

That was the split second my life could have changed but as usual, Fear triumphed. Instead of hearing her caring voice, it was Carl's harsh one that filled my ears with his threats of what he would do to me if I disobeyed him.

'No!' I almost screamed before turning and running away as fast as I could. I didn't wait for the bus, but ran the entire way home. In my room, I sat shaking on my bed and I opened my diary:

Dear Diary

You know I told you that Carl has forbidden us to have anything to do with Mum's family? That he shouted at us until we said yes? And Mum was crying all the time? I think she still is. So am I. I'm trying not to, I'm not a baby anymore. Today is the worst day ever. I did something really bad – Gran came to the school and I ran away. I hate myself for that. Do you think she'll ever forgive me?

Chapter 38

The following day, when I returned from school, Carl told me he had heard what had happened when my gran turned up. How had he known was the question that shot into my head. I thought that Gran must have rung and I waited for Mum to tell me that she had received a phone call from her very upset mother, but as usual since Maria's death, her pale face was expressionless and she didn't say a word.

'So, tell me exactly what happened,' my stepfather asked me. He must have known that it was the last thing I wanted to talk about. Not that he cared, he just grinned away while I tried to describe how I had clambered over the gate and run off. For me, it was one of the hardest things to do, but for him, it must have been one of his proudest achievements. He couldn't disguise his joy at the thought of me running away the moment I saw her, he loved the idea of making my grandmother upset. More than that, he loved how strong his control of me was becoming.

'Good girl, now tell me again,' he said, shooting a wide smile in my direction.

I could hardly bring myself to look at my mother, who sat there silently as he kept stopping me and asking questions as I went through every detail of that encounter. With every word that came out of my mouth, I wanted to cry in anguish while he on the other hand doubled up with laughter – 'Oh, I wish I could have seen her face! Well done, Emily! She did well, didn't she, Betty?'

No answer.

'Your family are not going to give up easily, are they, Betty?'

She shrugged.

He was right about one thing – they didn't.

Chapter 39

Carl might have congratulated himself on what he saw as his success in making us ignore Mum's family, but had he really thought what the outcome would be? Did he truly believe they would take it lying down? Because if he had, he got it wrong. They must have taken turns for our phone rang constantly. If Carl was home, the ringing tone placed a dark expression on his face.

'Leave it!' he snapped when he saw Mum begin to move towards the phone. 'We know who it is, don't we? It'll be one of your sisters or your mother.'

I don't know how many times she asked him to let her speak to them before she eventually gave up. She was too afraid to ring them herself because the first thing he did when he walked through the door was to check the 'last number called' facility. Other times, ignoring her, he would walk over to the phone and tell whoever it was on the line that Mum was resting or that Emily couldn't come to the phone because she was busy with homework before placing it down abruptly.

The family's next step was to call round when they thought Carl was out. He of course had anticipated that and made sure he arrived home at odd times so Mum never knew when to expect him. I don't know if she ever let them in, or what she said if she had – I just knew that she was not getting better from the depression that consumed her. At mealtimes I watched as she hardly ate and only spoke to agree lethargically with something he had said. Within a short time she had become a thin, grey shadow of the woman, who just a few weeks earlier had glowed with happiness.

But the one person Carl could not stop me seeing was Dad – he had a legal right, which he made very clear when my stepfather tried to put him off fetching me. It was the Saturday after I had run away from my grandmother that Dad picked me up from school. He waited until we reached the cafe before asking me what was happening.

'Your gran rang and told me about the other day after school. What made you act like that, Emily?'

Just remembering that afternoon made my eyes well up with tears.

He leant over the table and covered my hand with his.

'They're not angry with you, just terribly worried. So, what's going on with you and your mum?'

'She doesn't want to see them.'

'Why not?'

'Don't know.'

I gave the same answer to every other question he asked.

'I'm your dad, Emily, you can tell me anything,' he said.

Perhaps I might have believed him if we had not been apart until he obtained joint custody. It was during that time that I was brainwashed into believing he didn't care for me – a belief that however nice he was to me had not gone away completely.

My dad must have asked Lily to try and find out what the problem was for I had hardly taken my coat off when he made some excuse and disappeared, leaving us together. Lily, to my utter surprise, told me to come and sit next to her and asked how I was feeling, saying she understood it must be a really difficult time for me.

'You know, your dad is worried about you,' she told me.

Everyone was, it seemed.

'Emily, is there something bothering you?' she asked, placing her perfectly manicured hand briefly on my arm.

Don't trust her, whispered Fear.

'What do you mean?' I asked, desperately trying to buy myself a little time.

She lifted my chin then, so our eyes met.

'Is everything all right with you and your stepfather, is what I mean.'

Yet another Get Out of Jail card that I didn't pick up – it seemed throughout my childhood I was pretty good at ignoring them.

'Yes,' I managed to say.

'Are you sure?' she said, looking at me kindly.

At this my resolve almost disappeared and I nearly opened up to her. Nearly, but not quite, for Fear refused to remain silent.

You know she doesn't want you here, it muttered. *She'll tell your mum.*

An image of a pair of large hands with chunky rings shot into my mind.

'I'm OK, it's just that Mum is so unhappy and I wish Maria hadn't died, that's all,' I told her.

She didn't believe me, I just knew it.

Dad must have told her to ask me that. He should have asked me himself if he really wanted to know, I told myself rebelliously. But then I didn't take into consideration that he already had.

He must have thought that it might be easier for me to confide in a woman.

* * *

Seemed Lily was not the only female who thought I might open up to her. At school, the Head sat me down. At first, I thought she wanted to know how I was coping with my sister's death. By the end of our interview or 'chat', as she no doubt wanted me to think it was, from the questions she was asking I was pretty sure that my grandmother had been to see her – asking how often I saw Gran certainly gave me a clue. I guess she had told the Head that for reasons of his own, Carl was cutting everyone he could out of our lives.

Not that the Head was that straight with me. Instead, she asked how my mother was coping with the death of my sister.

'She's very quiet,' I told her, 'and very tearful all the time.'

'It must be a sad time for all of you, Emily,' she said, fiddling with her pen. 'And your stepfather?'

'Well, he's sad too.'

'Emily, I'm sorry, I should have asked how you are dealing with your loss and what it's like for you at home now.'

A difficult one, that.

I suddenly realised that I was not only twisting my hair, but sucking on my tongue as well – something I always did when stressed. Words had completely deserted me and I felt tears forming in my eyes.

Don't put your arm round me, I begged silently as I saw her move towards me – I would not be able to stop the sobs then. Instead, she just handed me a tissue.

'Emily, is there something you want to tell me? You know, anything said to me in here stays within these walls.'

Be careful, muttered Fear, *tell her you're just sad about your sister dying.*

So that's what I did. Not that I think for one moment she believed that was the only thing that was affecting me.

'I would like to talk to your mother,' she told me when she saw that I had totally clammed up.

'Why?' I asked, panic rising.

'Oh, nothing for you to bother about, just a routine parent-and-teacher chat.'

'She doesn't answer the phone,' I told her, but when I saw the concerned expression on her face, I wished I hadn't said that.

'If I give you the time I will ring, will you tell her? Just say it's nothing urgent and it will only take a few minutes.'

I agreed, though I felt as if a heavy stone had taken root in my stomach. Mum was bound to think the worst, that

I had told my headmistress something. Or, and another worry crept into my head, maybe it was my school marks she wanted to talk about. Either of those would result in me being punished. But I had no choice, did I? If I didn't pass the message along, the Head would ring anyhow and if she didn't receive an answer, she would no doubt write to her.

* * *

Once I got home, I saw to my dismay that Carl was already there. I had no way of giving my mother the message without him overhearing it.

'What does *she* want?' Carl asked impatiently when I told Mum the Head would be calling at five o'clock.

'I don't know.'

'Well, that's no surprise, is it? You never know anything,' he said cuttingly.

'She must have told you something,' Mum said, shooting me a worried glance.

Before I could say that she hadn't, the phone rang.

'You take it, Carl.'

'Don't be stupid, Betty! It's you she wants to talk to.'

My mother, seeing he was not going to move, picked up the receiver nervously as if it was a red-hot poker, not a phone.

That stone in my stomach grew even heavier as I heard Mum's replies:

'I see, yes.'

'I'll talk to her.'

'No, I can't think of anything.'

'Yes, we are all very upset.'

'Thank you for letting me know.'

'Yes, tomorrow afternoon's fine with me.'

'What did she want?' asked Carl and I noticed his knuckles whiten as he gripped the arm of his chair.

'She says she's concerned about Emily and wants me to go and see her.'

'You should have said you couldn't, that you're too busy.'

'I can't, Carl – she was pretty firm about it. She thinks Emily's depressed and her schoolwork is suffering, that she's clearly grieving over Maria's death.'

'Don't see why she should be, she never knew her. Just trying to get sympathy, aren't you?' he said, turning to me. 'Well, you can stop that nonsense right away! Taking advantage of what we're going through just to get attention. Now, look what you've done!'

Getting up from his chair, he lashed out with his hand, sending me staggering backwards. He just about snarled when he asked what else I had been saying to my teachers.

'Nothing,' I replied.

'I hope for your sake, you're not lying because if I find out you've been mischief-making, that slap's just a taste of what will happen. You understand?'

'Yes.'

* * *

In the end, they both went to the meeting the following afternoon. Just the thought of Carl being in the school talking to the Head made me shake with nerves.

When the bell rang, announcing that lessons were over for the day, I found them standing outside the classroom with the Head. There were warm smiles coming in my direction from all three of them. Mum actually put her arm round my shoulders.

'Home, darling,' she said in an artificially bright voice before thanking the Head for her time.

Before I knew what was happening, we were outside and in the car.

Nothing was going to be said until we got home, I realised. Not that either of them told me much of what went on in that meeting. Just that Carl blamed my gran – '*that meddlesome old bitch*' – for having to go in the first place.

'Why can't they mind their own business and stop interfering in ours? Saying Emily needs counselling and giving us a card with the woman's phone number! Means either the Head or your mother has already spoken to her. Next thing we know, we'll have Social Services knocking on the door – she's capable of that, all right, isn't she?'

Gran must have gone to the school for my sake. If she had guessed what the outcome of that would be, I'm sure she would have thought of another plan. I believe she had a shrewd understanding of what sort of man Carl was. Perhaps she wanted him frightened. What she could not have considered was what he might do to protect himself – use their 'interference' as he called it to move us to another area where we would not be known or know anyone.

He certainly acted swiftly. It took him just 48 hours to announce that he had found us a new house and we were moving at the weekend.

'Where is it?' Mum asked anxiously and I heard him name a town that was several miles away.

'And,' he added before either of us had a chance to say anything, 'no running around and telling anyone. Do you hear me, Emily? Don't you be yapping away to Ben because I'll know if you do.'

'But, Carl, that's miles away,' my mother protested before bursting into tears while I sat there, completely numb. I had allowed myself to hope that the disagreement between Carl and my uncles would blow over, that everything would be all right. But I knew when he told us about the move that nothing ever would be.

'Oh, stop that, Betty!' he snapped. 'We're moving to a better place and that's that! You should be pleased.'

* * *

That time is engrained in my memory, as is a small scar on my wrist. It's been there for a long time, a little faded over the years, but it never ceases to remind me of those last few days in the flat.

It was the day after he announced the move that my mother came into the bathroom while I was brushing my teeth. She leant over me, opened the small cabinet above my head and took out a razor blade.

'It's your fault, Emily,' she told me with blame in her eyes. 'All because of you we're going.'

She raised her hand and for a moment I was frightened it was me she was going to attack so I pressed myself against the wall. But I was mistaken there for she didn't even look in my direction. With horror, I watched as she raised her arm, held the razor in the air before bringing it swiftly down and slashing away at her wrist.

I remember so clearly how I screamed as she, without making a sound, dropped the blade into the washbasin. I couldn't move or speak when, her face expressionless, she held her arm as blood splattered onto the floor.

Hardly the right time for me to have a compete meltdown, but Fear never could remain silent: *You are going to be left living with Carl*, it said, and I opened my mouth and let my screams ricochet around the room.

No one can remember exactly what they go through when a meltdown is in charge of both body and mind. It's worse than any panic attack for the sufferer has absolutely no control over it. So I have no recollection of picking up that blood-stained razor, nor how, imitating my mother, I cut into my own wrist. Evidently seeing my dripping blood running down my fingers woke her from her stupor. I finally came back into the world to find my wrist bandaged and Mum, with a matching one, sitting near me on the floor.

Did she want to die that day? Did I?

I think for those few seconds, we both did. Or maybe we were crying out for help.

If so, our cries were never heard.

Chapter 40

I remember so well the day the furniture lorry arrived. It seemed to take no time at all for everything to be packed into it. First, the kitchen was stripped, then the sitting room and lastly, the bedrooms. Finally, several boxes full of our personal possessions were loaded on before the lorry doors were slammed shut.

I had been given my own cardboard box the day before, as had my mother. Our instructions were to pack our clothes and anything else we wanted to bring with us: 'Anything you leave behind will be thrown out. Understood?' said Carl. Much as I would have liked to leave the dreary selection of skirts and jumpers, I knew better. And I saw to my dismay that once I had placed some of those bulky garments in it, they were going to fill most of that box. I looked down at what I was wearing: were any of those things thinner than what was going into it? After removing my outer layer of clothing, on went the thickest shirt, jumper and skirt I had. Then I looked at my shoes and decided to wear the bulkiest ones. Perhaps that would gain me some space? I was disappointed to find that the space saving was minimal.

Where was I going to put all the books Gran and my aunts had given me, the drawings I had in folders and my collection of dolls from various birthdays and Christmas? Glancing around the room where all my possessions, except for the dolls, were arranged in neat piles ready for me to pack, made me summon up the courage to ask my stepfather for another box.

'No, Emily,' he said firmly. 'One is enough, so pack your clothes. Those are the important items. And make sure you put all of them in – you won't be getting any new ones if you forget anything.'

That was the end of that conversation and seething with resentment at his refusal, I went back to my bedroom.

Into that box I pushed down more clothes and the rest of my ugly shoes. There was one colourful item I came across: a hat my gran had knitted for me, brown with bright yellow bears stitched into it. A lump formed in my throat when I picked it up. Even now I can still remember the day when Gran, her face wreathed in smiles, slipped it onto my head – 'That will keep that busy little brain of yours warm,' she had said as she tugged it into place.

Carl had given a derisory laugh when I walked in, wearing it proudly. 'Makes you look even more of a simpleton,' he said scathingly. 'Take it off and don't ever embarrass us by wearing it outside again.'

Knowing his view, I tucked it under my navy-blue and grey skirts carefully. No way was he going to tell me to leave it behind! To me it was like holding a little token of the love she had put into every one of those stitches.

Next, I turned my attention to my dolls. Each one reminded me of the person who had given it to me. And often when I lay on the bed looking at my collection, I conjured up pictures of those happier times before Carl entered our lives. In my mind I saw all my birthdays where Gran would have baked a cake and I, in an effort to blow out all the candles, sucked in all my breath before letting it out in the biggest burst I could muster. 'Now make a wish,' I was told and closing my eyes and crossing my fingers, I did.

Not that I could tell anyone, I whispered to myself, *because then it wouldn't come true, would it?*

And now I can't remember a single one of those wishes so I don't know if they did or not. What a shame I had no clue as to what my future might hold, or I might have asked for those days to last forever. After the candle-blowing and the wish-making, one by one, an assortment of brightly wrapped packages was handed to me and smiling faces watched as I undid them.

There was one doll I had named Maisie, a flaxen-haired, blue-eyed one, wearing a sky-blue dress and holding a cream handbag. Just looking at her brought back the memory of the last Christmas my parents and the family had spent together. My mother would take me first to Gran's, where presents were given, and then we would all make our way down to my aunts' houses. There were my cousins of varying ages delving into their Christmas stockings while my aunts made breakfast for everyone.

'Just a light one,' they warned, 'we've got a big lunch to eat.'

Then there was the huge, sparkling Christmas tree, so tall it almost touched the ceiling. At its base were the piles of presents that, unlike our stockings, were not permitted to be opened until after the breakfast things had been cleared away. I'd never seen so many helping hands clearing the table as on that day.

After our lunch, when the adults were too full to move, all of us younger ones went outside to burn off some of our excess energy. I have a vague memory of family games being played later in the day, and of slabs of homemade Christmas cake, with its thick crust of marzipan and sweet icing, being passed around. By the end of the day I was drifting off to sleep and I know Dad had to carry me out. My parents must have put me to bed, for I seem to remember that I didn't wake up until the following morning.

Now those days were gone and Carl wanted to throw away everything that reminded me of them. Good memories, like old photographs, might fade over time, but they never vanish completely from our minds. Like an album of old photos, we can run through them in our heads and smile whenever we see them. We can almost taste the birthday cake and smell the needles of the pine tree.

Chapter 41

Standing in my room that day, it was apparent there was only a little space left in that box, just enough for one doll. I had to choose which one was going to come with me. *Take Maisie*, my inner voice told me, and carefully, I removed her from the doll family, wrapped her up carefully and placed her in the cardboard box, ready to go on her journey. I felt those treacherous tears – you know, the ones I kept telling myself that only babies had – form in my eyes at the thought of what I would have to leave behind. Carl clearly didn't want me to have room to take anything my relatives had given me, not the books nor my drawings. I had to choke back sobs when I looked again at my doll collection: it was as if they already knew they were going to be abandoned and their bright shiny eyes were asking me why.

My mother suddenly appeared in my room and without saying anything, started to fold my clothes. Even the ones that I had already packed, she took out and refolded before repacking them again. She must have seen my hat, understood why it was so precious to me and decided not to mention it.

'There, that gives you a little more room,' she told me when she had finished.

She glanced at my row of dolls – a couple had come from her and Dad. 'He's going to take them all to the hospital,' she told me, 'for the children's ward. They will make some sick kids happy.' That cheered me up, as did her unexpected act of kindness.

The last thing she did before leaving my room surprised me even more: she gently took hold of my arm, removed the bandage and peered at the cut underneath.

'That bandage can stay off now,' she told me. 'Not much more than a deep scratch, really. Good thing I keep a first-aid kit in the bathroom though. And Emily, don't ever try that again, will you?' She looked me straight in the face when she added gently, 'You will have a future. You're getting excellent school marks and one day, you will walk into a world that will be good to you.'

Before I could say anything in return, she walked away, leaving me wondering if I had imagined the expression of remorse on her face when our eyes met.

If I hadn't, it was a long time before I saw it again.

I wondered how she really felt about the move. Carl had told us it was a much bigger place and just needed some work doing to it, which he was arranging. I over-heard, as was my wont, him let slip the area it was in to Mum and lodged it into my mind. In my room, I looked it up on the map.

Not too far away, but far enough for us not to bump into anyone we knew.

Yes, Carl had got my mother and me exactly where he wanted us. In just a short time he had removed not just Mum's support group, but mine as well. Because of his timing, he knew when he did this that she was vulnerable and incapable of making decisions and needed her family more than ever. On top of that, he was taking her to a place where isolation and loneliness would become her constant companions.

There was no way Mum could arrange behind his back to meet up with old friends. Carl controlled the money that came into our house and exactly how every penny of it was spent. There was nothing he did not check, including each of her shopping bills. Every week I had seen him studying the receipts, which amused me because it took him so long. Out came his calculator and he punched in every total shown on the slips of paper laboriously.

Once, I couldn't resist asking him if I could do it for him. I loved seeing the look of fury on his face, which he wiped off quicker than it had appeared.

'Mind your own business and don't talk nonsense!' he snapped. 'Can't you see I'm busy?'

At least he did not show his annoyance by lashing out at me physically. A small victory, but small ones can all add up to a larger one in the end, can't they?

Chapter 42

The morning we finally left, the three of us climbed into the car and Carl drove behind, slowly following the furniture lorry.

That day I said goodbye to the housing estate I had lived on for nearly five years. Goodbye to all the youths rolling up and down the roads on their skateboards before, with arms outstretched, they mounted the base of a wall. I could hear the click of their heels against the concrete, followed by whoops of excitement as they spun off again. I said goodbye to the teenage girls who, in their tight, short skirts, were cheering them on, and goodbye to the children's playground, where once I had spent all my spare time.

As we drove through the estate I noticed for the first time how time had taken its toll. Paint blistered by the seasons was peeling off window and door frames, net curtains hung drably from windows and most of the small, square-front gardens were overgrown with coarse grass, weeds and dead bushes.

Naturally, Carl made his usual derisive remarks about the louts, the sluttish girls and the rundown houses in those overbearing tones of his. He said he was happy that he was taking us away from it. But still, it had been my home and I had seen it as a friendly place where people with kind faces smiled and waved at me when I walked to get the bus to school or to the local shops. As we drove out of the estate, I turned to look out the back window and said a final goodbye to it as well.

I should have said goodbye to my cousins.

To my aunts.

To my uncles.

And to my gran.

For I never saw them again.

I also should have bidden a farewell to my childhood for it ended that day.

Part Two

Chapter 43

If I felt down in the dumps when we left, the weather seemed pretty dismal too. A thin winter sun peeked through the thick clouds hanging in a dull grey sky. Once we drove off the highway and onto the country roads, the trees, without their canopy of green leaves, were just dark, sombre shapes, their out-flung branches casting shadows over the windy road we were travelling on. Fields waiting for spring to change their dark muddy soil into crops of green and gold stretched either side of the road. The only colour I could see came from the thick evergreen hedges hiding country estates.

I spotted a signpost with the name of our destination town on it and knew we were almost there, wherever that was. Before we entered, the furniture lorry and our car turned left onto a road where rows of new-build houses of various sizes stood behind low white walls. My mother looked hopeful when she saw them, while I guessed that our new home was not going to be there. I was right – we drove past and then turned down a rutted lane. At the end of it we came to a square, squat, single-storey stone building, with small windows and a dark blue door.

'We're here,' Carl told us, pulling up behind the furniture lorry.

'What, we're going to live here?' my mother said and I heard no hint of pleasure in her voice.

'Why, Betty, it's ours. I bought it,' he said. 'I told you it needs a bit of work doing to it – I've got a couple of boys coming over to give me a hand this week. Won't take us too long before it's looking great. Now, out of the car, both of you. Oh, and see all the land around it? That's ours too.'

'The land' being an overgrown garden at the front and when later I went out to explore what was at the back of the house, I found a vegetable garden where not much looked alive. However great the building that resembled an outhouse more than a home might look in the future, it certainly did not look it then. Things did not improve either when Carl unlocked the door with the largest key I had ever seen and we all walked into a small, dark hall. Even the furniture delivery men looked slightly aghast at the amount of grime and dust we saw in each room we walked into as Carl showed them where to put everything. The sitting room was now termed 'the lounge', I noticed, while 'my study' was the title given to a very small box room. And I really don't want to dwell on how awful the kitchen was – my shoes just about stuck to the floor.

The moment the delivery men had gone, out came scrubbing brushes, disinfectant and bleach. Gallons of disinfectant and bleach were poured into the toilets and wiped over the bathrooms before we tackled that kitchen, which took us the entire day.

'Think the pigs must have lived in here,' my mother muttered as she emptied yet another bucket full of greasy water.

'It was rented out for a while,' was Carl's only concession when asked how it had got into such a state.

Mum didn't mention that it would have been a very good idea to have got a team of cleaners in before we moved there, nor did he offer any explanation as to why he hadn't.

I was told to put my things in a small room at the back of the house. This, he told me, was where I would sleep until he had finished smartening the rest of the house up. The only good thing about it, I thought, was at least I might not hear their rows as the room was the furthest away from them.

My mother managed to produce a couple of scrappy meals during the day and then it was bedtime. Going to my room, even though it was an uncarpeted, airless place that smelt of damp, was still a relief.

Dear Diary
I don't like it here. The house is so ugly and dark. Mum's not happy either. And we are both tired out from cleaning. I helped as best as I could, but it still looks horrid. And I miss everyone so much.

Chapter 44

I have said that my daughter is wired up a little differently, a little more differently than I was at her age. What I, my close friends, my partner and in-laws see is a loving, lively little girl.

What other children see is someone who is not the same as them.

And it's that difference that invites bullying from her peers.

I can't explain that she should ignore the ones who jeer at her. Nor can I get through to her what it is she does that appears to encourage them. She simply wouldn't understand and would probably think I was angry. Maybe if she looked different, the parents would sit down and explain to their children that we are not all the same and that they should be kind to those who are not like them. But Sonia looks like any other five-year-old – a bright, alive little face, a wide smile and boundless energy.

She so wants the other children to play with her. It just about breaks my heart when I see her gaze longingly at groups of children laughing and giggling together. I know she's hoping that one of them will walk over and invite her to join them in their games.

This is something that never happens, though.

I'm aware of the reasons that they turn their backs on her. Her wanting to be liked makes her mimic them. If they laugh, she laughs too; if one falls over and cries, she does as well, and if they scream out when high on a swing, she opens her mouth wide to release the same sound, even though her feet are still firmly on the ground. Already forming their herd instinct, the others huddle together to cast out the one they see as being different. Should she try and approach them, at best they turn their backs; at worst, they push her away and shout aggressively.

It's not the first time when I have gone to collect her from school that I have found her sobbing. Yesterday, the teacher had not brought her out to meet me, which always meant something was wrong.

Her eyes were still wet with tears when I walked into the classroom. She was sitting by her teacher, a kind young woman who had her arm around her. I bent down and gave her a cuddle while I listened to another story of her being mocked.

Of course, like any mother, I felt the urge to march up to those bullies and lash out at them and not only with words. Instead, I kept her hand tucked in mine as I took her home.

Her sister, still wobbly on her feet, tottered over and put her arms around her. Sonia smiled up at me then, everything forgotten – she was back in the place where she knew she was loved. Watching them together puts a smile of content-ment on my face. It also springs open another drawer, the one labelled 'First Day at My New School'.

*   *   *

The following day, Mum took me to the new school. Carl had already left for work so there was no chance of him giving us a lift. Instead, we walked up that lane and caught a bus. Doubtless once she met the Head, my mother would manage to talk about my clumsiness, as well as point out some of my issues with food and a few other little things. In other words, make sure the school knew I wasn't quite normal right from the start, just in case they didn't notice.

'Mind you pay attention on the way,' Carl had said the night before. 'Then you'll be able to find your way home, won't you?' I could tell by the offhand manner he men-tioned it that he was not particularly concerned about me getting lost.

'Yes,' was initially all I could muster, not, 'Oh, I'll just draw a map in my head on the way in and refer to it when I come back.' Not something that would make a good start to the day, for he always grew angry when he refused to accept that there were some things I could do that he was incapable of. 'I'll write down a couple of the road signs,' I added none too nonchalantly, but acting the part he liked.

A child who didn't know that much and had to turn to her stepfather for help.

Mum, I noticed that morning, had actually put on a little make-up, washed her bobbed blonde hair and sorted out a pretty deep-blue woollen dress to wear under her stone-coloured mac. I was a split second away from telling her she looked pretty when, without drawing breath, she told me to finish my breakfast, that she had a lot of work to do and walking me to school was a one-off – I'd better pay attention on the journey because she wasn't going to make the trip twice, did I understand?

My compliment disappeared from the tip of my tongue almost as quickly as it had appeared.

The first sight of the school, yet another grey stone building behind iron railings, made me feel completely lost. The playground was already teeming with children who clearly all knew each other. Outside the gates, a group of women, who must have met at the school gate twice a day for months, stood chatting. Other children arrived by car and ran excitedly into the playground, calling out to their friends as though they had been separated from them for weeks.

No one spoke or smiled a welcome at us when we walked past the group of mothers to the gates. They appeared too wrapped up in their own conversations to notice us. My mother did not seem to be any more comfortable than me. She took hold of my elbow firmly, squared her shoulders and walked us briskly into the building. Looking back, I realise that in a way, it was her first day too. Her first in walking past groups of people where she didn't know a soul and her first at talking to a headmistress she had never met before. After all, she had grown up in the town I had spent all my early years in. Her family were well known in the community and we seldom walked down a road there without being greeted by an old school friend or someone she had worked alongside. Making small talk to strangers was just not something she had any experience of.

Luckily, she didn't have to ask directions to the Head's office. Dressed in a smart tweed suit, a tall, dark-haired woman with horn-rimmed glasses was standing by the door as we entered. Her welcoming smile removed the initial impression of the severity her clothes gave her, as did the warmth in her voice when she introduced herself as Elizabeth Dunn, the Head.

'Ah, Mrs Corby,' she said, stretching out her hand. 'And you must be Emily,' she added, smiling down at me.

'Now, Emily, we have your school reports from your old school. I know you will find some of the classes a little different, as you are joining them mid-term, but looking at the grades you achieved in your last school, I'm sure it won't take long for you to catch up. Now, why don't I take you to your classroom and introduce you to your teacher?' she asked before she and my mother said their goodbyes.

That was the friendly part of my first day there.

The teacher introduced me to the class and I felt a flush sailing up my cheeks as what seemed like 20 pairs of eyes looked me over. I had noticed on my way in how most of the girls were dressed. Pretty coloured jumpers and skirts just above their knees. No clumsy shoes for them either – they wore ballet shoes or neat leather lace-ups. Most of the girls in my class had long hair tied back with a ribbon matching their outfit. Mine in contrast was even shorter than the time the hairdresser had cut it. Mum had been instructed to keep that style in place and she had managed inexpertly to retain the shortness, if not exactly the style. It looked as though a small pudding basin had been sat on the top of my head before it was trimmed with blunt garden shears. Well, that's what I saw when I looked in the mirror anyhow. I could feel all those eyes sliding down from my hair to my below-the-knee skirt until they finally rested on those clumpy shoes and thick grey socks. I must have stuck out like a sore thumb and judging by the expressions on their faces, I was sure there was no doubt in their minds either.

Still, the teacher seemed nice enough as she introduced the lesson – English. Staring down at the books I'd been given, I could see they were different from the ones in my previous school. But the subject was the same, the usual spelling and grammar. I bent my head down while hands shot up in the air to inform the teacher they either had a question or an answer to one of hers. Mine stayed still in my lap – I had no wish to draw any attention to myself.

The next lesson was Maths, which I soon found out was to be a difficult one. My previous teacher had accepted that I worked out the answers in my head. This new one made it clear that he wasn't going to. But with more complicated Maths, it was beginning to become a problem. There were no signs of my working out the numbers, not even a few little squiggles – I just wrote down the answers.

'And how did you come to those answers?' asked the Maths teacher.

'I worked them out in my head,' was the answer I gave. I could hardly say in front of the class that just looking at the questions sent the answers to my head, which in turn forwarded them to the fingers that wrote down the answers.

When I first started learning simple arithmetic and the times tables I had no idea that the answers came to me in a different way from all the other children. But before I was seven, I had learnt that was how it worked for me. Another reason for me to be labelled weird, though then it was said with some degree of affection.

'Well, that's good. All of them are right, by the way,' he told me. 'But one day, you will be sitting important exams and they will want to know how you worked out the answers. The examiners will fail you if you don't show them how you have reasoned the Maths so make sure you put down all your working-outs, all right? I believe in marking everyone's work the same way as they will when you go to the senior school so that means you get much lower marks if you don't do it the way the teachers expect you to. And you don't want that to happen, do you?'

Of course, the answer to that was 'No, I don't.' Facing Carl with a less-than-perfect school report would lead to him punishing me.

I nodded, but I knew it was going to be a problem. I had never really understood just how my brain had worked everything out, that was the real issue. I could probably manage to show some of the workings-out, but not all of them. I had a sinking feeling that as the Maths became more complicated, the problem would only get worse and I wondered if there was a way I could slow my brain down and see how it got to the answers – something I had tried more than once but with no success.

By the end of the day, I had the titles of a couple of books I needed to read, some Maths questions to answer and an essay, or as the teacher had called it 'a story' about what we did at the weekends. This, I knew with some certainty, I would have to make up – I could hardly write, 'Try and avoid Carl as much as possible'. I decided to conjure up a nice memory and so I described a day when I was at one of my family get togethers. Now that would work – I just altered it a bit to make it sound as though it happened most weekends.

All that day I had tried to switch off my inclination to draw comparisons with my old school, where I had felt popular with both classmates and teachers. I already knew that it was going to be different here. On our lunch break, a couple of girls asked me where I had lived before we moved and then wandered off to join their friends as soon as I told them. No one in the playground showed any interest in my joining them – their little cliques were already formed and they clearly did not want to enlarge them. Unless another new girl, with dreadful clothes and a terrible hairstyle, came into our class, I guessed I would be stuck on my own for a very long time.

Might as well read on the breaks, I decided, perching myself on a wall. I expect that got me a lot of stares, but by then I didn't really care. If they were not going to be friendly, I would carry on doing things my way. For me the important thing was to do well in the end-of-term exams otherwise there would be trouble at home – I knew Carl would make no allowances for a new school and a curriculum change.

At the end of my first day, without any goodbyes coming in my direction, I took myself home. Neither Carl nor Mum thought to ask how my day had gone. Instead, my stepfather told me he had put an alarm clock by my bed set for 7:30am – my mother needed a lie-in and I was old enough to make my own breakfast. Now that was a plus – I wouldn't have to see him the moment I left my room.

* * *

I woke to a freezing-cold morning and shivered as I looked out of the frost-encrusted windows at the grey sky and decided it was unlikely to get much warmer. After hastily swallowing a slice of toast, on went a thick sweater over my vest and the thick navy-blue skirt I hated underneath my raincoat. To keep my head warm, I pulled on the hat Gran had knitted for me.

Shivering must have stopped me thinking straight because if I had, I might have worked out that it would have been a good idea to remove that hat before walking into the playground. Then I would not have been subjected to the whoops of laughter that broke out when I appeared, nor seen fingers pointed in my direction.

Once I realised that it was me who had caused that mocking laughter, I had a flash of memory of another conversation with Carl before we left our flat: 'The school I have arranged for you to attend will be better for you,' he had told me. Meaning, I understood perfectly, *You will be on your own there. No cousins to protect you, no friends to spend the break with and no Ben still wanting to get you home safely. Even better, no interfering grandmother watching how I'm treating you.*

Then I had wondered just how bleak my life could get.

Now I knew.

I was never going to fit in there.

Don't show them they bother you, said Reason, my inner voice. *Hold your chin up and ignore them.*

So, I did.

Chapter 45

What can I say about the following years? I worked hard at school, ignored my classmates' mocking jeers about my eating habits and other peculiarities as best I could. In contrast, I was praised by my teachers and at the end of every year, I came first again.

At home, I learnt to cope, up to a point, with Carl's unpredictability while counting the days until I could escape to Dad's. I had my diary to confide in, although I did not write down all the details of every beating, every hair pulling, every taunt and every act designed to humiliate me.

Had I done so, they would have filled every one of my diaries six times over.

The worst of the beatings occurred when I was still in junior school. It was when my first school report came in, the one I thought I was so clever in altering. Carl was by now used to me being first in my class. He expected no less *'after all that work he had put* in' when I *'knew absolutely nothing'*. I had been given a low mark in Maths but a high one in English. In other subjects I was close to the top, but not first. Although the teachers had written glowing remarks about how well I was doing, that would not impress him.

I just about shook with fright when I saw the report, knowing he would not be happy. And when my stepfather was unhappy, he took out his frustration by punishing me. I hadn't been beaten since the move – oh, a few slaps here and there, but I had learnt to handle the pain of those – so I guess I was due and those grades would play into his hands all right. The teachers' comments about how hard I had worked were not going to cut it. I knew that he took a perverse delight in me not living up to his expectations and really enjoyed ridiculing me, holding anything with mistakes on it up in the air and waving it about. Once satisfied that I appeared sufficiently cowed by him yelling enough insults to work up his temper, those big, hard hands of his would lash out.

I just knew the beating would be bad. Anything connected to my education brought out the worst in him. My anxiety levels grew so high that I began getting panic attacks, which started around then and have refused doggedly to leave me to this day. When they come, they keep me awake most of the night, I'm so afraid of the nightmares sleep will bring. Unreasonably, I believed that during those unwelcome spells, closing my eyes would mean that I would wake to the worst-case scenario.

It was during those early hours when my brain was swirling around that I made a plan: I would alter the grades on my report. After crawling out of bed and picking up Tippex in one hand, a calculator in another, I got to work. I made the grades a bit higher – nothing unbelievable, just enough to hopefully save me. And I used the calculator to ensure the averages worked together. My stepdad wasn't one to miss out on detail like that – I knew he would double-check it.

I worked all night and for some reason it never occurred to me that a report full of Tippex might look suspicious – I was only nine, after all. As you can imagine, I got caught. Instead of tackling me, he rang the school. Told the Head he was a little unsure of the report I had given him and he would like to compare it to the original.

He and Mum went to see the Head. I don't know much about the conversation, just that she didn't understand why I had done that – my grades were good for someone who had started their new school in the middle of term. And that's exactly what she told me when I was summoned to her office. She said Carl and my mother had just left and told me the reason why they had been to see her. Each word that came out of her mouth caused the icy fingers of Fear to run down my spine.

She didn't appear to be angry with me, more concerned than anything else when she asked why I had tried to change my report. I gave my stock answer to that question – an embarrassed wriggle on my seat, followed by 'I don't know.'

'Your stepfather seemed concerned that you had done it because you didn't want to disappoint him. I told him your grades were very good for someone who had started midterm. Didn't you read all the comments your teachers wrote?'

After I told her that I had, I could feel her waiting for me to say something more. She was far from satisfied with my answers, I could tell.

'Emily, is there something bothering you, something you've not told me about?' She wanted to know. And as others had done over the years, she looked me straight in the eye, waiting for an answer.

'I miss my friends at my old school,' I managed to say.

'Of course, but you'll make new ones here soon.'

Not going to happen, they think I'm weird.

Not that I let those words escape my mouth. I realised that she was now watching my fingers twisting my hair.

'Your stepfather appeared very understanding. He told me he's helped you with your homework more than once. I understand that he did not come into your life until you were five. So, how do you get on with him?'

Again, those piercing eyes looked straight into mine.

Don't say anything, whispered Fear.

'Oh, fine,' I told her.

She let me go then after telling me to have more confidence in my ability before finally adding, like my headmistress before her, that her door was always open and if I had a problem, to come to her. It was so tempting to say that I was frightened to go home and then ask the Head to phone my dad and tell him to come and take me away from that ugly house and Carl. So, what stopped me? Knowing each step I took towards home was a step nearer the thrashing in store for me.

Perhaps if I had had some coins in my pocket instead of the bus pass Carl had bought for me, I might have gone into the red phone box I passed, just might have made that call. But I hadn't, and trembling, I jumped straight onto the bus. My hands were still shaking as I pushed open the front door. For a moment no one spoke and I stood frozen to the spot as the two of them stared at me. The atmosphere in that room was thick with menace.

Run, screamed Fear, *run as fast as you can! Get away now!*

For once I did not stand my ground and wait for the outcome. Instead, I turned around, pushed myself through the front door and headed for the lane.

He caught me, of course he did. His fingers grabbed hold of my coat then spun me round and slapped me hard. There was a stinging pain as the rings cut into my face and I felt a trickle of blood sliding down my cheek.

Oh, God, I thought, *he's left them on.*

'Where do you think you're going, Emily? You've nowhere to run to now, have you? No Gran to take you in!' It was the sound of him sniggering as his hold tightened that made the hairs on my neck stand up. I just knew I was in danger; this was a side to him far worse than anything I had seen before.

'We're going in now.' Clenching the collar of my coat tightly, he shoved me up the path and back through the front door. 'You've disgraced your mother and me!' he shouted with spittle flying into my face as he shook me so hard, my teeth just about rattled. 'You useless little cheat! Thought we were stupid, did you? Well, we'll see about that when I've finished with you!'

I was numb with terror when my bladder let me down and there was nothing I could do to stop myself peeing.

'You filthy little slut!' he roared as he drew back his fist and drove it hard into my back, just above the kidneys. Pain flooded my body as more blows rained down until my legs buckled and I fell to the floor. My ears were ringing and through a fog, I could hear my mother screaming, 'Stop, Carl, for heaven's sake stop now, you'll kill her!' I felt his breath as he crouched over my body. His hands were around my neck, squeezing it tighter and tighter, as with black dots floating in front of me, I gasped for air.

I heard Mum scream again. I don't know how, but I have a memory of her hands grasping his shoulders, trying to prize him away from me. But she must have realised then that her husband could no longer hear her, he was beyond reason.

I could hear ringing in my ears as I began to lose consciousness and then a sudden stream of ice-cold water hit my head and those hands finally fell from my neck.

'Don't move yet,' my mother's voice warned and as my sight slowly came back into focus, I could see her leaning over me, still holding an empty bucket. 'I'll help you into your room.'

'Carl, sit down now,' she said, turning to him. Amazingly, dripping water as he moved, he obeyed her and sank into his chair.

Mum helped me up, took my arm gently and guided me slowly to my room – but not before I had seen the glazed look on Carl's face.

Yes, he had lost it all right.

Gingerly, my mother helped me undress and brought in the usual medicine and gently rubbed cream on my bruises. She also gave me something to help me sleep, which worked almost straight away.

In the morning she appeared as my eyes opened, her face white with worry and dark shadows under her eyes.

'You can't go to school this week,' was all she said.

Which meant more excuses had to be made up for the school.

Which one would it be? I wondered.

Flu, chicken pox or whatever illness she could think of would explain my lack of attendance.

It was when I went to the bathroom and glanced in the mirror that I understood why I was not going to be let out of the house. A dark ring of bruises wound round my neck, I had a swollen black eye and a cut cheek where one of his rings had struck me. Just looking at my reflection made me feel sick and dizzy, as did the fact that my whole body throbbed with pain and I could hardly stand.

I stayed in my room for three days. Food was brought in (not that I had any appetite), more lotions placed on my bruises, and most of the time I slept. The one thing my mother insisted on was for me not to flush the loo when I peed. I didn't understand why then, but now I do – she wanted to check for blood after that hard thump to my kidneys.

After the third day, she tried to make excuses for him. I can't remember what they were for I blocked the words from even entering my mind. He didn't say he was sorry either. Apart from the odd glare sent in my direction, he mostly ignored me, which was precisely the way I liked it.

My mother didn't just phone the school, she actually went in, ostensibly to pick up any work I needed to do.

Talk about covering all bases.

Chapter 46

It was not long after I recovered from that beating that I discovered my mother was pregnant again. Not that she was glowing with happiness as she had done before. But then there were few signs of Carl bestowing presents on her, or making her feel special either. I seldom saw her spend time putting on her make-up anymore or rushing off to the hairdressers. Nor did I hear him telling her with a wide smile that he had arranged a special day out for her and suggesting she had better change into something more glamorous, as he had not so long ago.

I no longer heard her giggling or saw her looking up at him, doe-eyed, when they shared a private joke. Nor did I see him putting his arm around her, or patting her on the knee or on the behind. Not only had all the sparkle gone out of my mother, it had also deserted their marriage, it seemed. That did not mean that he never hit her – I saw the bruises on her arms, the dark shadows under her eyes. She must have been aware of the times he slid into my bedroom too.

Did she really not care? I asked myself.

If she did, to the best of my knowledge she made no effort to stop the abuse even though she must have known what he was up to in there.

* * *

There were days when the atmosphere in the house made me extremely uneasy. It was as though we were all walking on eggshells, just waiting for something to happen. I tried to escape by spending as much time in my room as I could. Homework was always a good excuse. Not that it stopped me having to eat with Mum and Carl and clear up afterwards. Nor did it put an end to my household chores, which increased at the weekends. Duties that Carl always inspected closely after I had finished, hoping to find a smidgen of dust or a neglected ring around the bath – in fact, anything that would tell him I had left something undone and cause him to yell at me.

Another of his warped little games was to decide which one of us was out of favour with him. It was as if he wanted an audience, be it only of one, when he made his choice of which one of us to pick on. I had come to loathe being in the same room as them for when it was my mother's turn, he would cross-examine her as to who she had seen, who she had spoken to on the phone, even which shops she had visited.

'No one,' was the answer to the first two questions and 'You've seen the receipts for the shops I go to, haven't you?' to the last one.

In contrast, he would then show me some degree of affection. After practically reducing Mum to tears, he would pay me some compliments, praise my schoolwork and tell me I was becoming rather pretty. While we all like praise, I cringed at his. He succeeded in making me feel even more uncomfortable, especially when I noticed how his eyes would shift in my mother's direction to gauge her reaction to him being friendly to me.

There was one evening when he was all smiles and told me that soon I would have a better room, one where I would be more comfortable when I did my homework.

'I'll put in some bookshelves for you as well,' he added. 'I know how you like reading, it's next on my list of things to do.'

For the first few months we had lived in the ugly house, his free time had been spent *'getting it just right'*. Which meant that it had just been transformed into a larger version of the flat, though even more oppressive. Talk about the darkness in him being reflected in his colour schemes! Burgundy made an appearance everywhere again, as did splashes of dark gold, and as for that heavy solid furniture he liked so much, it really managed to make the place even gloomier if that were possible. Let's just say there was not one attractive feature in the house, not one part of it was bright and cheerful. Carl seemed to think it all looked wonderful though. Personally, I thought it resembled Dracula's castle.

I have often wondered if my stepfather had any regrets about what he had accomplished for there was no sense of happiness in our home. You know the expression, 'Be careful what you wish for', closely followed by the warning, 'Lest it all come true'? In Carl's case he might have had a clear idea of what it was he wanted, but had he ever thought of the outcome? The feisty woman he had met and married was gone for good and the child he had tried to both shape and control did not love him. And underneath all of his blustering and arrogant ways, did a seed of fear not take root and tell him one day I might just talk? For in spite of all his slandering of my father and how much he tried every which way to make me doubt Dad's reasons for seeing me, Carl had never quite managed to complete that last step – to separate me from him.

Chapter 47

I started noticing that while I was getting ready for school, my mother would make a dash from her bedroom to the bathroom, where it seemed she stayed for a long time. Pausing outside a couple of times, I could hear the sound of her retching. Then, when she emerged, I saw her face was a pasty white. She was definitely not well, I decided, and shared my concerns with Dad at our next meeting.

He always asked after Mum and this time he also wanted to know whether her depression had lifted at all – 'Is she getting back to her old difficult self yet?' I heard remnants of a former affection in his voice but he seemed never to ask when Lily was in earshot – I can just imagine what her reaction might have been.

I told him that I wished she was looking better. But no, nothing much had changed, although she no longer stayed in bed for the whole morning or sat staring at the walls without saying a word.

'She still takes those pills though,' I said.

'And Carl, how's he coping?'

'Carl's the same as always,' I said, not going into any details before steering the conversation back to Mum.

'I'm worried about her,' I told him. 'She always seems tired and she has huge dark shadows under her eyes. And now she's throwing up every morning as well. What do you think is wrong with her?'

'I think she's most probably pregnant again.'

'Well, she's not mentioned it and I've not heard them talking about it either.'

'Maybe she doesn't want to say until she's had a scan. What happened last year was terrible for her, she must be so afraid that it could happen again. But if you're worried, Emily, why don't you just go and ask her?'

'Yes, OK, Dad, I will,' I answered doubtfully for I was not someone she ever seemed to want to talk to. She hardly acknowledged my presence when she saw me in the morning or when I returned from school. Not that I told him that.

* * *

On the Monday morning, I decided to ask. At least then I would know if my mother was ill or if there was a baby on the way. I waited until she came out of the bathroom before blurting out my concerns: 'Mum, are you being sick all the time because you're going to have a baby?'

'Yes,' came the answer but without the smile that had lit up her face just over a year ago.

She sat down in the kitchen looking, if anything, more tired than ever and told me that she was going to see her old doctor – 'I know Carl won't be pleased with me going to my hometown, but he's been my doctor for years and before him, it was his father. I just don't want to go to one I don't know.'

I could tell she was not far from crying then.

'I won't say anything,' I promised, feeling some warmth at her confiding in me.

'Don't go mentioning anything to Carl, will you?'

'You mean he doesn't know about the baby?'

'Not yet.'

Chapter 48

Mum didn't tell me what the doctor had said, or if it was going to be another baby girl. If she had gone to her GP and had one of those photos, she would have known, wouldn't she?

I don't think she cared either way.

This time I felt no excitement, I almost felt sorry for a child coming into our world. I thought of that time when my mother was pregnant with Maria and how happy she had been and how excited I was too. But neither of us had those feelings when she carried Mark, my baby brother.

The months leading up to her giving birth were completely different to the time before. Carl no longer strutted around looking proud – without Mum's family, he had no one to impress, had he? He still appeared not to have any family of his own. There were no visitors bearing gifts of handmade baby clothes, no excited aunts on the phone congratulating them both, no Gran dropping in with homemade food and no more sisterly lunches for Mum to look forward to. The only difference to her lifestyle, which mainly consisted of sitting around looking depressed or cooking, was that she refused to touch alcohol. Not that my stepfather took any notice – he continued drinking enough for both of them. In the years since he had moved in with us, he had gone from being a man who watched his diet and was a moderate drinker to simply sloshing it back. Now, excess flesh had settled on his stomach and jowls and he no longer looked like the trim, fit man he once was.

To begin with, I had heard my mother try and persuade him to go a little steadier. Glaring, he had brought up her family – how many beers they sank at those get togethers, how he never touched a drink before six o'clock and what about all those pills she popped? She was not to insinuate that *he* was the one with a problem.

So, that was the end of her trying to reduce his intake – it was also the end of her trying to stand up for herself.

Carl might have denied he had a problem, but I saw him waiting impatiently for the hands of the clock to tell him it was six o'clock. That's if he was at home and not out with his business friends, which was happening more and more.

Even though Mum and I were quite often left alone for most of the evening, we never slipped back into the closeness that had meant so much to me. I so wanted to go back to that time just over a year earlier when I had rested my hand on her stomach and felt the ripples of tiny feet kicking. Or share my smile of happiness when, flushed with excitement, she showed me those photos from her scan.

Mind you, that little tadpole-like creature was nearly lost even before it had created a bulge in my mother's stomach. She told me one evening when we were alone that it was thanks to my actions that the baby was still where it should be. If she had told Carl about being pregnant then perhaps she would not have come so close to miscarrying. Her excuse for not confiding in him was she was so afraid of losing the baby. If that was the reason, those fears nearly came to fruition.

Haven't I already said that I felt as though both my mum and I were walking on eggshells? The atmosphere in the house was by now making me feel uneasy and I disliked being in the company of them both.

There might not have been much conversation between Mum and I, but that didn't stop the tension between us – a tension Carl had skilfully orchestrated. Even during those times when he behaved like a normal husband and stepfather, neither of us was fully relaxed. Family meals could be pleasant for several days on the trot and then my mother's cooking was praised. Not that she ever looked pleased with compliments as she once was – I suppose they never quite made up for the many complaints that Carl spat out at her when he was in a foul mood.

Those other occasions, or should I say the majority of times, he took a delight in quizzing one of us about how we had spent our day. He would use every trick in the book to trip us up so that he had an excuse to inflict some type of punishment. Not knowing which one of us he was going to choose to question set our nerves on edge, a situation that made us both understandably selfish. It was a relief for the one who was not chosen, who instead of receiving barbed comments mixed with unrelenting questioning was the recipient of warm, friendly smiles.

Nearly always the questions were about Mum's family, the 'enemy' as he saw them. Since they had been cut out of our lives, Carl had not just rewritten history, he had actually come to believe that they were all set against him. There was no reasoning with him on that subject, so neither of us tried. Had we contacted them, he would ask one of us. Caught a bus and gone to see them? Had they come over here? All of which we vehemently denied – after all, it was the truth.

Even worse than those evening meals was the apprehension we felt when, knowing he had been meeting his friends, he was due to arrive back late and probably drunk. Both of us were aware that the slightest thing could make him fly into a rage, but when he was worse for wear from too many gins, there was no knowing what might set him off. I had gradually learnt since we moved house that alcohol made his moods unpredictable. It was as though it had a voice of its own, telling him how to act. Sometimes it told him to be soppy and loving towards one or both of us, other times the voice told him the opposite.

It was the opposite that frightened us.

Would he arrive clutching a bouquet for 'my beautiful Betty' or might there be a scowl on his face as he looked around, searching for anything he could blame one of us for? Those were the thoughts uppermost in our minds as we sat on high alert, waiting for the sound of him coming through the door. By then, my whole body was tense, my mind full of dread as to what might happen. Would he find something I had done wrong and, one by one, slip those rings off before punching me? Or would this time be my mother's turn? Not that I had ever seen him hit her, just heard the sounds. That was until the one evening he came swaying in, long after his dinner had gone cold.

Just one look at his flushed face set off warning bells in my head. *Could I quietly disappear into my bedroom?* But no, seeing me trying to wriggle off my chair, he placed himself in front of me.

'Oh no, you don't! You stay here, got some questions for both of you. First, though, where's my dinner? I'm starving!'

Mum just told him it was a fish pie and that it would not take long to heat up as she quickly placed the dish in the microwave. I wondered why she stood watching it circling and then realised it was to stop the question she knew was coming. Once she heard the ping telling her the meal was warm enough to eat, she laid it on the table and throwing a teabag in a cup, made herself some tea.

Apart from the scrape of cutlery as he piled his plate high and the sound of him chomping away, the kitchen was heavy with an ominous silence I would have done anything to escape. But I knew that if I made any movement, even asking permission to go to the toilet, he would grab hold of me and force me back in my chair. For some reason he was determined I should stay there to see and hear everything that was about to transpire.

'Well, Betty, what did your mum have to say when you met up with her?' he asked once his plate was scraped clean.

Where had that come from? I wondered as I glanced from him to my mother, lids lowered, and saw her back stiffen. I guessed that somehow, she had found the money to escape the house and take herself off to see her old doctor. *But had she seen her mother as well? If so, just how had he found out?* I got the answer to that a couple of seconds later.

'You've been a little careless, haven't you?' As he held out his hand, I saw a bus ticket lying in his palm.

'It's not mine,' she muttered. 'I don't know where you got it, but it's not mine.'

'Wrong answer! I found it in your coat pocket, so it must be yours. Or is it Emily's?'

His glare swivelled around in my direction.

'No, I haven't been anywhere, only school and I have my pass anyhow,' I protested.

'Come on, Carl, leave her alone! She's not got the money to catch a bus out of town, has she?' Mum suddenly said. 'Anyhow, I know where she is all the time.'

Now that was a first, Mum sticking up for me – I shot her a grateful look.

'Oh, I'm sure she has money tucked away. Don't tell me you don't scrounge money off your dad: money he should be paying us for your keep. Still, that's interesting, your mum says she knows where you are all the time. Strange, seeing as you've been going to some girl's house after school, haven't you? Does she know about that?'

My voice quavered as I tried my hardest to defend myself: 'It was just once – we were walking up to get the bus together after school, that's all. And she wanted me to stop at her house so she could show me her new puppy, I promise that's all.'

'And what have I told you?'

'I'm to come straight home.'

I waited for him to make a move in my direction, but his anger was not directed towards me, it was Mum who was his target and I could see her hands were trembling.

'Did you know about this, Betty?'

'No.'

'It's up to you to be stricter with her, to make sure she obeys my rules. But then, doesn't look like you've been doing that either. So, tell me, who did you see, Betty, when you went off visiting?'

'Carl, let me explain . . .'

But he told her he wasn't interested in explanations, he wasn't really in a listening mood, especially as far as excuses were concerned – he just wanted the truth.

'Carl, I can explain . . .' she repeated.

She just wanted them to sit down on their own, she pleaded next. I could tell by the way she was twisting the edge of her jumper in her hands just how nervous she was. I also realised that she was desperately trying to think of something that would stop him losing his temper.

Just tell him, Mum, I felt like shouting.

I could hear her voice quake as she repeated that it was not what he thought it was.

As the words left her mouth, we both found ourselves looking at someone we scarcely recognised. Oh, I had seen my stepfather losing it before, but this time the mask of fury slid over his face was even more frightening than when he had beaten me so badly. For a second none of us moved, then a bellow of rage tore from his throat, his arm drew back and he hurled the dish with the remains of the pie at my mother. She ducked and it flew above her head, hit the wall and shattered on the kitchen floor. Pieces of fish pie and vegetables slid down the wall and oozed onto the tiles. She seemed almost frozen with terror as her husband leapt from his chair. His large hands, which after his third gin the night before had lovingly stroked her waist, now grabbed hold of her, lifting her a foot into the air until their faces were almost touching. Just as he had done with me, he shook her hard before dropping her onto the floor. Not that he was finished, this was just the warm-up. He bent down from the waist, twisted his fingers into her hair and clenched his fist. It would be seconds before his fist would punch her hard and once he began, there would be no stopping him. In desperation, I flew at him and, clutching hold of his jacket, screamed at him to stop. He tried to push me away as though I was no more than a tiresome flea, but I refused to let go.

His eyes were empty as he turned and met mine.

'She's having a baby!' I shrieked as I pummelled his chest with my small fists. 'A baby, Carl!'

Finally, I had found words that reached him. His hands fell to his sides and he shot me a look of disgust.

'Is that true, Betty?'

'Yes,' she whispered.

'So that interfering little bitch of yours knows this and I don't?'

'She heard me being sick and put two and two together, that's all. I went to my doctor to have it checked, that's why you found the ticket. I wanted the same one I had last time, he knows what happened before. That's why I went to him. And he was the only person I saw.'

At this she burst into tears, her shoulders heaving with sobs.

But he made no move to comfort her, no apology either. He just looked at us both with those cold fish eyes.

'You better get this mess cleaned up, Emily,' was all he mumbled before stalking out of the room.

* * *

I'm not saying peace reigned in the house after that. There were a few improvements, though mostly offset by Carl enforcing stricter rules.

- I was to come home straight after school. Mum was to check the time when I walked through the door and write it down. He had worked out exactly how long it should take me.
- He would give me a list of all my duties and I was to make sure that they were all completed – Mum was to check that.
- He wanted to see just how much homework I really had, so I could not use that as an excuse not to help around the house.
- Not only was I limited to home and school during the week, but at weekends, apart from the times when I met my dad, I was to stay within the boundaries of the house and its garden – 'You've enough to do here, what with your homework and helping your mother,' he told me.

  Meaning: even if you were able to make friends, I wouldn't allow it.
- Finally, when he was home, I was not to speak unless spoken to.

Rules were also laid down for my mother. She must have obeyed all of them, for during those months of pregnancy, I didn't hear him shout at her once or notice any new bruises. Not that the same could be said in my case. He accepted the fact that she needed to rest and mustn't pick up anything too heavy. Like the vacuum cleaner, for instance – which meant my duties increased. He insisted she register with a local doctor – that visit to her old GP was to be the last one.

As he had done in those last weeks at the flat, he started returning home at unpredictable hours. Each time he walked in, he would check the last call made and received on the phone.

Every day he was at the door, waiting for the postman to arrive. Regardless of what type of envelope it was, the postmarks were closely scrutinised before he slit them open and examined the contents thoroughly. Did he really think that there would be letters to us disguised as an electric bill or a reminder about paying the TV licence?

When it came to shopping, that could be done once a week, he told us. So, there was no reason for either of us to go to the shops. He would drive my mother to the supermarket – after all, she should not be carrying any bags. Meaning even short trips into town had to cease.

My classmates might have been looking forward to their summer holidays but I just wished that the school remained open seven days a week, all year round.

I dreaded to think just what plans my stepfather would have for me during those weeks off school. To make matters worse, Dad had told me that he, Lily, baby Crystal and Paul were going camping for several weeks during the summer. He rang Mum to ask if I could join them. Naturally, Carl refused categorically, insisting I told Dad that I did not want to go away while my mother was pregnant.

I decided I had to show I had things to do for school that would give me the excuse to stay in my room as much as I could, so I went to each of my teachers and asked them to give me as much homework as they could for the holidays. From my English teacher I asked for a written reading list so Mum could get the books from the library. I hoped that borrowing these books would therefore appear compulsory to my mother and Carl.

The teachers all looked pretty surprised at this request, but they all agreed smilingly. Unfortunately, one of them told the class about my diligence and what a good example I was. Imagine the derisive mocking comments that caused. Now, I was not only weird, I was an even more unpopular teacher's pet. Let's just say when school broke up, I did not receive a chorus of friendly goodbyes, more like a few well-aimed taunts.

Ignore them, said Reason, which was easier said than done. I missed the friendliness of my previous school, desperately missed my cousins and hated the thought that for the next six weeks the only faces I was likely to see belonged to Carl and my mother. But, as I walked slowly through those gates as my fellow pupils called out to each other, whooping with joy that the holidays had begun, I came to realise that true loneliness is having no one beside you when you are in a crowd.

Chapter 49

Carl did not wait long for my revised list of duties to be handed to me. First, he asked for details of the homework I had been set for the holidays. Luckily, he did not know that apart from recommending a couple of books, at our ages none had been given – 'Doesn't look like much, does it?' he said as he flicked through some of the pages, 'Gives you plenty of time to still do your chores.' He made it clear that those chores were to be finished and inspected by either Mum or him before I could take myself off to my room to study.

I noticed that vacuuming everywhere had now been added to my list of weekend duties. And he had also written all the others down, just in case I had forgotten them: dusting all surfaces, cleaning the bathroom, cleaning the kitchen and on the daily list was setting the table, washing up, keeping my room tidy and ironing my own clothes.

Doesn't sound too bad, I decided, and it wouldn't have been had my stepfather not seen his opportunity to create another game – one where, if he won, I got slapped very hard.

But what was fun for him wasn't quite the same for me.

* * *

Carl tested his new game out in the living room. With its heavy dark furniture, it was the most overcrowded room in the house. Although my mother never voiced an opinion in regard to interior design, I don't think she liked it any more than I did because if he was out, we both ate in the now-renovated kitchen. Even though the tiles in there were burgundy too, the cooker and work surfaces black, it was still lighter than the living room and the dining area. When my stepfather was home, he demanded his evening meal be served on the large oblong table that sat under the window. And of course, he expected it to be laid properly as well. That room was his pride and joy, so he was definitely going to inspect it carefully once I had finished cleaning.

'Right,' he said, rubbing his hands together on the first Saturday of the holidays, 'you can start in here. I want every bit of furniture moved so you can also dust underneath after you've vacuumed. Then once you've done that, put it all back in its rightful place.

'Every single piece, Emily, understood?'

Of course I did, he just wanted to make cleaning the room as difficult as possible.

'And,' he repeated, 'make sure everything is put back exactly, and I mean exactly, in the same place.'

So, what did he do to ensure that it was? Why, he measured up the spaces they occupied, of course. He wrote it all down in a notebook – table so many centimetres from wall, chair so many centimetres from table, and so on. Then when I was finished and had used all my strength to push the heavy furniture back where it had been, he would appear. Out would come that metal tape measure and round every piece of furniture he would go. It took him ages to check and double-check just how many centimetres out it was.

One centimetre equalled one slap, two and he hit twice.

I tried the next week to place small markers where the table legs had stood, but Carl must have guessed I would do something like that and giving me that smirk-tinged smile, he picked them up and placed them in his pocket.

Luckily, Dad had not gone away for his holidays yet. When we met, I asked him to buy me the same type of tape measure as Carl had. He was a bit curious about that request – I just told him it was part of a school project when he asked, which seemed to satisfy him.

Before the furniture was moved, I also measured up every item and noted it down in my head – not having to write it down was a true asset. Without seeing me clutching a piece of paper, he wouldn't be able to work out how I did it; the metal measure I placed down the back of my skirt.

* * *

The following Saturday, my plan went into action. I had already measured up everything the day before, when he was out. Once I had finished, in he came with that metal tool of his, which he liked flicking in the air.

Round he went – twice.

He was not happy.

I was, though.

He glared at me – I'd obviously spoilt his fun for the day.
No excuse to hit me.
Carl loved his games.
And I loved beating him at them.
Another small victory chalked up to me.

* * *

It was near the end of that summer holiday that I finally said hello to Mark, my blond-haired baby brother. Having produced one son who was healthy, Carl didn't waste any time getting my mother pregnant again.

A year later, she gave birth to her second son, Robert.

It was also during that year that I walked through the doors of my senior school. And it was there that I finally got a glimpse of the world that one day I would belong in.

The senior school I was to attend was not much further away than the junior one. It was larger, with a well-stocked library, which was the extent of my knowledge. Like the junior school, uniforms were not worn. I wished they were, then at least I would look the same as everyone else.

I had asked my mother if I could have a couple of dresses in lighter colours and a pair of prettier shoes. Her reply was a sigh: 'Pretty clothes for you are the least of my problems,' she told me. She did agree that I needed a couple of teen bras as my body was beginning to change though.

So, there I was on my first day, walking into the school where the new girls were already in their chosen groups. *Not much changes then*, I thought when no one lifted their eyes, smiled and greeted me. Looking around, I recognised some of the pupils from my junior school, others I had not seen before. I suppose like some of my previous classmates, they had been friends in their junior schools. Most probably some had even known each other since their mothers met in antenatal classes and had gone to the same baby and mother groups – a group that Carl hadn't wanted my mother to join.

'What, at your age, Betty? You'll look more like the boy's grandmother! Don't think that's a good idea, do you?'

Of course, she didn't – not after that remark anyway. It was not mentioned again. Nor was the subject of my having clothes that would help me blend in with my peers ever brought up. The long and the short of it was I wore another dark coloured plaid dress, well below the knees, and a pair of those sensible shoes I hated when I walked through those school gates for the first time.

*　　*　　*

All around me I could hear the chatter of how the summer holidays had been spent. The voices of the posh, confident ones, who with their deep tans and new clothes were the loudest. They were busy saying with much waving of arms and giggles how wonderful Spain, France or Greece had been. How their days had been spent on the beach, the food in the hotels was amazing and as for those Latin waiters, weren't they just gorgeous? More giggles and eye-rolling would accompany those remarks.

Not much point in me trying to join in then, was there? Even if it wasn't holidays they were talking about, it would be the new car their father had ordered, the latest music or how their mother took them shopping for new clothes because they had all grown so much over the last few weeks. I never heard any of those girls talk about their home being a council flat or how they had moved into a place that was just about falling down. Nor did I hear them moan about their mums choosing their clothes – I guessed they didn't. From the snippets I overheard, they chose their clothes themselves and their mothers just whipped out a credit card. So even if I had approached them, just what could I have talked about anyway? Make-up and pop stars seemed to be the other popular subjects, but I doubt if housework, looking after my baby brother and how good I was at dusting would have been.

Or I could make a long list of all the things I had never done. Never gone on one single holiday and never eaten in a restaurant where gorgeous waiters took my order. Don't think a teashop with my dad would count with them either.

It was the lunch break when one of those girls turned to me. 'Nice dress,' she said and just for a moment I felt a flush of happiness, thinking maybe they were going to be friendly to me. Big mistake for when I said, 'Why, thank you,' and smiled at her, her whole group rolled their eyes and snorted with laughter. Without saying another word, the girl turned back to her friends.

Was she happy that she might have made me feel crushed, a nobody not worth talking to?

But she was wrong for I had toughened up over the two years I had spent in junior school. I simply took out a book, found a wall and sat on it.

Ignoring them, I found, transferred the power to me.

When it came to lessons, I was surprised none of the girls I had known in junior school were in the same class as me and very few of those gleaming, confident ones either. I also noticed that there were more boys than girls in my class. I had been placed in what was called the A stream – one for future high achievers. The Head had explained to us that morning in assembly that although the exams that would help determine our future were several years away, it was still important that we kept them in mind. 'Some of you will want to go on to further education,' she told us. She went on to explain that there were scholarships available for children who had succeeded with high marks in their exams and the word 'university' was mentioned for the first time. This made my ears prick up – they were places students could live in, weren't they? My 11-year-old self decided, *I'd better work hard and go to one, or how else can I get away from home?*

It was an ambition that I failed to confide in my diary, because that evening, I truly believed I had learnt about something that I could put in action far sooner.

Chapter 50

Dear Diary

A children's helpline was advertised on television today. It's all part of an organisation called Childline. You should have seen my stepdad's face when it came on – never seen him move so fast to turn the TV off! But not before I had memorised the number. I just have to wait till I see Dad and get some money for the phone call.

Those people will tell me what to do and I can't get in trouble if I talk to them. They promise that they won't make a phone call and tell my stepdad or Mum what I plan to tell them – that he beats me really badly and when he comes into my room at night, he touches me in places he shouldn't and I hate it. I hate the feel of his hands on me.

I've decided I'm going to run away after I speak to them. They won't make me go back, will they? I already know what I will pack in my bag when I leave and one of the things will be you.

* * *

The evening that I shared those plans with my diary, my stepfather had switched on the TV to watch the news. He had already plonked himself down on his chair, a second or third tumbler of gin wrapped in his hand, before he realised that he had switched on a programme about Childline, a children's charity – 'Don't want to listen to that rubbish,' he said, jumping up to switch it off, but not before I had heard enough to understand what that organisation was all about. Their phone number, which I promptly lodged in my mind, had flashed onto the screen a second before he turned it off.

I felt Mum's eyes glued on me – she had seen that number come up too. From the worried expression on her face, I saw when I eventually glanced in her direction, she was pretty certain that I had memorised it. Carl might refuse to believe that I could retain whole pages of books in my mind so storing a phone number would be pretty easy, but Mum knew I could. It was one of those things that made her uneasy around me. She would also have a shrewd idea that once in my room, I would mull over the words she and I had both heard – *touching, inappropriate behaviour, frightened* and the most important one, *confidential*.

Mum must have been scared stiff that I would find a way to make that phone call. She and Carl needed to find out fast if that was my plan. I mean, they could hardly ask me outright, could they?

Now, who might I confide in? Not a human – I had no friends because they had made sure of that. Not any member of my family either as Carl had manipulated their disappearance from our lives, so all that was left was my diary. He and Mum already knew about all my thoughts and the problems I had written neatly in it. They were right to think that as soon as I was in my room I would unlock it and out would come the pen my stepfather had given me – because that's exactly what I did.

* * *

It only took me until the following day to discover there was more than one key to my diary. No wonder I had been given one each year. And there was I, thanking Carl for what I had felt was a thoughtful present – silly, naive me. When, after returning home from school and walking into the living room, the first thing I saw was the bright shiny key on the coffee table and next to it my diary – my *open* diary, the one with whom I had shared all my private thoughts.

It was pretty obvious that they were no longer private.

Sitting on a chair closest to it was Carl, wearing that mocking smirk I so detested. I glanced at my mother, noticed there was no smile on her face – if anything, she appeared listless, but then she was not someone who lived in constant denial as her husband did. She would have known just how serious it would be if I went ahead with the plan I had written about on those pages. Not only would there have been social workers asking questions and police arriving at the door to question my stepfather, she would have been implicated as well.

Not that I understood all of that then. If I had, I might not have been so afraid of their reaction. Carl placed a finger on the damaged journal and turned it round so that the red lines and exclamation marks he had added were clearly visible. I could see my last entry had been torn out.

'Well, Emily, I've just been doing a bit of correcting for you. If you're going to write insults and rubbish like this in the presents I've given you, at least get the grammar and spelling right! Your mother gave me a hand with those corrections, didn't you, Betty?'

'Yes, Carl,' she said in a voice devoid of any animation.

Still unaware it was them who should be frightened, I could hardly move, far less speak. After the journey home, I wanted to go to the loo – I didn't want another accident like the last time my bladder let me down.

'Got to go,' I blurted out and before he could stop me, I managed to get my legs to work and rushed to the bathroom. Not that he let me have any peace, even for the short time it takes a young girl to relieve herself.

'Don't think you can hide from me in there!' he shouted through the door and I felt those familiar fingers of icy terror returning.

Going to be bad, muttered Fear.

Best get it over with and try not to let him see how scared you are, said Reason.

The mistake I made was thinking that what I had written about him would make him angry. *Wrong!* He enjoyed knowing how much I hated what he did to me – it all added to his feelings of power. He had read everything, knew how much I hated his actions, how much I missed my family and how, without my old school friends and cousins, I was finding school difficult. He now knew so much about my doubts and my secret thoughts, but none of that was as bad as the last entry I had written, which he had ripped out.

'When you've finished in there, you come back to the sitting room.'

He said it calmly through the door, for where else could I go and there was no lock on my bedroom door? The calmness of his voice frightened me even more – it meant that he had planned exactly what he was going to do and I didn't know what it was.

'Sit down,' he told me when I walked back in. Cautiously, I placed myself nearer my mother than him. Not that I expected her to stick up for me, I was just a little further away from his fists there. 'Now, explain what made you write all these insults about me and your mum that are in here, Emily.'

I tried to find some words that might work as an explanation, but I really couldn't think of anything.

'Cat got your tongue, has it? Well, let's take the bit where you blame me for you not seeing your gran. What have you to say to that?'

'I miss her, that's all.'

'Well, I doubt she misses you, especially after you ran off that day. You think she's forgotten that?'

'No,' I agreed miserably.

'Got that right! Now, you also wrote how you miss that smarmy Ben too. And you think he would want to see you again now? You made it clear that you didn't want to speak to him too, didn't you?'

'Yes,' I murmured.

'Now, you've written that you're going to run away. See-ing as you've upset so many people, where exactly do you think you're going to run, eh? Your dad's perhaps? Where Lily doesn't even want you playing with her daughter? Oh sorry, your *half-sister*. I don't think so, do you? Have you forgotten he's the man who chose to take the television rather than his daughter? No doubt he lied to you about that because that's what your dad does – he lies. And you should know that by now. After all, you were the one who caught him shagging that scrubber Lily, weren't you? And she wasn't the only one!'

I tried to block my stepfather's voice out as he went on and on, repeating all the insults about my dad I had heard so many times before. The sound of his hectoring tones was beginning to make me feel incapable of thinking for myself. He waited until he could see I had no defence left in me, that I was just about drooping with exhaustion, before he brought up the final part he had read – my plan to phone Childline.

'So, let's go back to your last entry, shall we? Now, I want you to listen very carefully to what I have to say. I'm the man who took in someone else's child, put a roof over her head. Your mother could hardly afford to find her own place when I met her and your dad wasn't helping, was he? It was me who sorted everything out for you both. I even helped your mum get that job. And look what I've paid out for you . . .'

He went on to list everything I had needed over the years since he moved in with us – clothes, shoes, books, bedding and . . .

The list seemed endless.

'So, who do you think paid for all those things?'

'You,' I whispered.

'And why have I sometimes had to smack you?'

'When I did something wrong.'

'Exactly! And when I come into your room and give you a cuddle, what have you written here? That I was doing something filthy to you! And that you were going to report me and get me into trouble. Well, let me tell you this, Emily, no one would believe I was anything but a caring stepfather. Mind you, they might suggest that a girl with your imagination and sordid thoughts should be put somewhere. No doubt you've heard of places where problem children are sent?'

I hadn't, but I nodded my head anyhow.

'Now, is that what you want?'

'No,' I said and I could no longer stop the tears cascading down my cheeks.

'All right then, we'll talk no more about this. Oh, and take your little journal with you – it reads better now.'

At this, I gulped – I had expected a thrashing at the very least, but he was far too clever to lay a hand on me.

Not that time anyhow.

I guessed no more diaries would be coming my way, not that I wanted one now. I felt angry with myself for being so gullible – why on earth had I believed that I was the only one with a key? I placed the ones I had been writing in for so long in a box. It wasn't the diaries' fault that I had been hoodwinked. Sharing my thoughts with each one of them had given me great comfort. What was I going to do now? Without a soul I could talk to, I needed some way of expressing myself.

It was about a week later that I had a brainwave. We had started studying French at school, a language that I had really taken to. I found it easy to master the accent and spent time learning new words every day from the French–English dictionary. I was pretty sure neither Mum nor Carl could read one word of it. All I had to do was find out – simply ask them if they could check my spoken French from a book because we had a test coming up.

First, I asked Mum: 'No point asking me, Emily, I never managed to learn it at school. I thought it was a waste of time,' she told me.

'What about Carl?' I said. Thinking on my feet, I then threw in a bit of flattery. 'He knows so much, doesn't he? I expect he learnt it at school and was good at it.'

She looked a little surprised – saying nice things about Carl was not something I did very often.

'I'll ask him,' she told me.

Asking Carl if he knew something he clearly didn't quickly put him on the defensive.

'No, I don't speak any French – that's for Nancy boys to learn!' he spluttered.

Meaning you were useless at it.

'And what are you wasting your time for anyhow? Learning a language you'll never have any use for. You're not likely to go there on holiday when you leave school now, are you?'

Yes, I am.

'No, of course not,' I answered. 'I agree with you, it's a waste of time. Still, at least it's not Latin, but' – and here, I managed to look a little nervous – 'I don't want to get bad marks, do I?'

'I suppose not, just don't waste any more time than you have to on it. There are other, more important subjects, aren't there?'

'Yes, of course,' I answered meekly.

Good, I thought, *he can't read a word of it!*

* * *

The following weekend, I was due to meet Dad and I would ask him to get me a couple of ordinary exercise books that I could turn into my private journal and a pen – I didn't want to write with the one Carl had given me anymore.

When my stepfather snooped in my room and looked inside those simple lined notebooks, he would believe what I had told him – they were just school projects. *Best make them appear to have been marked as well,* I thought, placing a packet of gold stars on my list. *Now, he'll be completely fooled,* I thought with a grin.

I put my plan into action the next time I saw my father – I told him I was in the A stream at school and needed some extra notebooks and a new pen. Apart from congratulating me on doing so well at school, he didn't say anything more. He took me into WH Smith and told me to sort out what I needed and to choose a good pen. And if there was anything else I needed, just to tell him. He didn't even raise an eyebrow at those gold stars when he paid.

I must say over the time I wrote in my diary, it really helped me come first in French.

> *Dear Journal*
> *So good to have you back with me. I know you don't look as smart as my diary but it makes no difference, I will like you just as much. You are my secret, the one he will never find out about.*

The next entry in that journal, as I had now renamed it, was not so upbeat. I had gone back to the original plan the Head had spoken to the class about – getting to university. I wanted to see what Carl's reaction would be. For some time, I had felt his continuous put-downs were because instead of being pleased with all my good marks, he was beginning to resent them.

I'll put it to the test and if he doesn't like the idea, he'll have forgotten all about it long before I finish my schooling, I thought.

When I had the chance, I casually dropped in that my teacher had told me I was university material. I did wonder if he would appear pleased and then manage to take all the credit because of all those months of home schooling I had endured. But no, his brows lowered. A scowl appeared on his face as he questioned me relentlessly. The first question was 'Who was the teacher?'

'Mr Davis, my English teacher.'

'And what made him say that? Trying to get round you, was he? Asked to stay on for some extra work once school is over, is that it?'

'No,' I said and I started to feel uncomfortable.

Just what was he suggesting? That Mr Davis was the same kind of man that he was?

I quickly told him that I was not the only one Mr Davis had said that to – he had brought it up with several of us.

'Why not the whole class?' he persisted.

I told him that the whole class had been asked if they were hoping to qualify for further education, but only a few of us had put our hands up to say we were.

'And you were one of them?'

'Yes.'

'Oh, that explains it then, he was just being nice. It's not as though you're likely to get a place, is it?'

'I don't know, it won't be for years anyway,' I said quickly.

Now I knew that over the coming years he would try and stand in my way of applying to any university, so best I never mentioned it again.

'Well, let's forget about that. You just run along and do your homework. I've got something to show you later.'

'Later' meant when my two little brothers were in bed and my mother, exhausted from looking after them all day, had either fallen asleep in front of the TV or gone to bed.

Which of course left him free to creep into my room. *'Later' was not a word I liked.*

* * *

Dear Journal

I don't know how to tell you this. He showed me some pictures in a magazine, women with no clothes on. I didn't know that hair grows down there. And there were really ugly men putting that horrible thing into where the hair is – I wanted to be sick.

I don't want to grow up and have to do that. He says everyone does and I'll love it when I'm little older. And then he told me that's how babies are planted in their mummies' tummies. I sort of knew that, just didn't want to think about it. I do want a baby, even two or three, when I grow up. I wish I had a big sister I could talk to – I feel so muddled now.

It was several magazines he had brought into my room while I was trying to read a book. Knowing he was going to turn up at some time or other had made concentration hard. When he slid into my room and I saw he was just holding some magazines, I actually thought for a moment that he had bought them for me and gave a sigh of relief – a sigh that quickly changed to a gasp of shock and disgust once I saw what they were. The lurid covers were bad enough, but when he flicked them open, I wanted to shut my eyes.

There was picture after picture of naked women with huge breasts, sitting with their legs apart, showing those parts that are meant to be covered.

'Nice, aren't they? Wonder if you'll look like that when you're all grown up.'

I'd rather die.

Then he opened another one and I began to feel sick. There were men getting on top of the women, with that horrible red thing going inside them.

'Please,' I said, my face burning, 'I don't want to look at them anymore.'

'All right, that's enough for your first time. But you think you're beginning to grow up, don't you? All that silly talk about university . . . Well, grown-ups like this sort of thing. You'll find out if you go out into the big world.'

He must have been proud of himself.

He had just found another punishment for me.

Chapter 51

I have realised for some time that I am fluent in three languages. The first two are French and English. The third one, I had learnt by the time I was seven: it is the language of abused people. This language is so secret, only those who have been abused can speak or understand it. Why? It's because our brains work differently from those who have had a secure upbringing. We tend to over-analyse everything, but it's that which has kept us mentally alive or perhaps the word should be 'sane'.

It has given us the strength to become survivors. To refuse to live the rest of our lives with the word 'victim' stamped on us for all to see. Although when we meet one another, without saying anything, we can recognise each other. We are the ones who have been trained to look carefully at every single detail of our lives and surroundings. When we meet new people, we have to weigh up whether or not they are trustworthy, for trust is not something we have in abundance. Why would we, when as children, we stayed awake at night dreading the sound of footsteps outside our bedroom doors?

And our mothers, who were meant to make us feel secure and loved as soon as we came into the world, betrayed us. Instead of building our self-confidence, they turned a blind eye to what was happening when we were small and help-less. And then, when we felt trapped by our dependence as we entered our teens, they withheld any advice as to how to deal with our changing bodies for by then they had come to see us as their rivals.

So, when we meet new people, we look for anything that will tell us who the real person behind the smile and show of friendliness really is. We take in every detail – their body language, how they move, how they sit, certain words they use, expressions flickering across their faces when they think no one is looking, how they laugh and at what, and who their friends are.

All those tiny details most people ignore, we analyse. How mad is that? But that's how we decide who to tread carefully around and who we let into our lives. It's also how I recognised another one of us.

Her name was Marion and she was the first friend I had made since we moved. The tentative friendship I had for a short time with Cindy, the girl who had taken me to her home to show me the puppy, dwindled out in a very short space of time. Not because I wanted it to, but because I was not allowed to bring her home.

'No,' said my mother when I asked, 'you know Carl doesn't like you ignoring your homework.'

'Can I have her over on Saturday then?'

'No, Emily. Carl is home then and you know he wants peace and quiet.'

That's one way of describing his shouts if either of us upset him.

The next time I brought up Cindy's name, it was to tell my mother I had been invited to her ninth birthday party.

'That's the same weekend you go to your dad, isn't it?'

'Yes, but he could pick me up from the party, couldn't he? He'll be pleased I have a friend. He's always asking me if I have made any at my new school.'

'Of course he does, means he has to spend less time with you, doesn't it? The answer's no, Emily.'

Cindy accepted that excuse, although she looked disappointed when I told her.

The next one she didn't accept.

She had asked me to come to her house for tea after school on the Monday after my return. 'I'll save you a piece of my birthday cake,' she told me.

'No,' said Carl when my mother mentioned it, 'you've got to concentrate on your homework. Don't want another bad report, do you?' he added mockingly, deliberately reminding me of the punishment he doled out when I had tried to alter my report.

I tried to explain to Cindy that I had to do my homework. She pointed out that we had very little to do in the juniors and I always got top marks anyhow.

'Just come for a little while, I've got your piece of cake ready for you,' she said pleadingly.

'I can't.'

'I thought we were friends,' she said tearfully.

'We are.'

'You never let me come to your house. My mum says it must be because your parents don't think we're good enough.'

That accusation completely silenced me – I could hardly say that Carl thought no one was, now could I?

She looked at me so hopefully, just wishing me to say something that would keep our friendship alive, but there was nothing I could tell her. Instead, I turned and walked away before she could see the tears in my eyes.

Cindy was the last person who tried to be friendly to me at junior school. She ignored me whenever we bumped into each other and now at my senior school, she was part of the confident girls' group. I wondered what she had told them. In the playground, I had seen her eyes swivel in my direction before she made some remark about me to her circle.

Chapter 52

My new friend Marion was different. She took no notice of those habits of mine which still made some students mock me. Like me, she kept herself aloof from the other pupils.

All I knew about her, apart from the fact she was skinny with a head of vibrant red curls and a freckly face, was that she hardly said a word in class unless she was asked a direct question. But there was something about her self-containment that made me feel I would like to know her.

'You're clever,' she once told me when we were walking out of class and I felt a link begin to form between us.

'Not really,' was my answer, 'I just have a good memory.'

'But that's what clever is,' she protested with a grin.

She asked me what I was reading on our breaks and looked amused when I told her it was a book on French grammar and that I was trying to learn a minimum of ten new French words a day. Not that I told her why learning French had become so important to me. Gradually we started spending our break times together, until after a couple of weeks she asked if she could come back to my house.

There was a silence between us for a moment when I tried to think of an excuse.

'They're strict with you, aren't they? Mine too.'

If Marion had not worked out just how strict my parents were, she was under no illusion after she witnessed me panicking when I spotted Carl's car parked outside.

'Oh, shit!' I exclaimed when we were just about to walk through the gates. 'It's my stepfather!'

'See you tomorrow then,' she said.

I was thankful that without being asked, she hung back so we no longer appeared to be leaving together. Later, I realised that she recognised why I didn't want him to see us together.

* * *

'Who was that red-headed girl you were talking to?' he asked as soon as I climbed into the car.

'Oh, just one of my classmates,' I replied as breezily as possible for I was aware that if he thought she was more than that, he would find some way of stopping the friendship. He seemed to accept my explanation and hummed cheerfully as he started up the car.

'Thought we could go for a drive,' he said and my heart lurched. There was no way what Carl had in mind would be just a simple drive, with maybe a stop for an ice cream. *And I was right.*

He drove out into the country until he came to a wooded area, not unlike the one that I had learnt to cycle in.

'Just want to chat,' he told me, parking the car under some trees. 'I've got a present for you.'

Please don't let it be more of those horrible pictures.

But no, to my surprise he took out a delicate silver chain from his pocket: 'Do you like it?' he asked.

And what could I say but yes, because I really did.

'Oh, I do, it's so pretty,' I told him.

He told me to bend my head forward so that he could do up the clasp for me.

'It's our secret,' he said. 'Keep it tucked under your collar.'

I must have looked completely astonished – this was hardly what I was expecting. He started chatting to me normally then and asked how I was enjoying helping Mum with my two brothers. A picture of the pair of them shot into my mind – chubby little Mark, who as long as I held his hands could already totter a few steps, and dark-haired Robert, who would clutch hold of my finger and give me a gummy smile when I came back from school.

'I like helping with them,' I said honestly with a smile. 'They're so cute and Mark's already trying to say my name.'

'I expect you will want children of your own one day?'

And I could feel his eyes watching my face, gauging my reaction.

'Yes, of course,' I answered and for some reason felt a little frisson of unease at that question.

He then brought up the subject that he always seemed to want answers to: had I thought what I might want to do when I finished school? I had already told him that I had university in mind. He had heard me, but clearly wanted to ignore it.

Tell him what he wants to hear, muttered my annoying companion Fear.

'Don't know really,' I answered as my brain scrambled around, trying to think of something that would please him. 'I thought if I do well in French, I could get a job as a hotel receptionist. Or maybe work with children – I'm getting experience with that all right!' And I managed to flash him a wide, beaming smile.

'Or have your own,' he repeated. 'We'll just have to wait and see what the future holds, won't we?'

'Yes,' I replied.

At this he gave me one of his warm smiles and I knew I had chosen the right answer. He then told me he thought a summer job might be a good idea for me over the next holidays – it would give me some pocket money and get me out of the house as well.

'How does that sound?'

I had to admit it all sounded pretty good to me. But that didn't stop my feelings of unease. Did he have a hidden reason for being like this? When I was younger, I would have taken him being nice at face value, but not any longer.

His next words aroused all my suspicions.

'You know I love you, Emily, and only want what's best for you.'

You've got to be joking!

'I was drawn to you the first time we met. There you were, all big-eyed and innocent.'

Well, thanks to you, I'm hardly that now.

But I had learnt enough over the years to humour him so I nodded at his remarks, thanked him again for the present and told him I would not take the chain off as it was so special. That seemed to work and apart from my knee being patted a little too high up for comfort, he just drove me home.

What had he really been up to? I couldn't help but wonder.

Over the next couple of years, this question would gradually be answered.

Chapter 53

I was a bit embarrassed when I met up with Marion on our morning break. Not that I needed to have been. She was her usual friendly self and made no comment about my stepfather and the fact she had worked out why I didn't want to be seen talking to her. Instead, for the first time she talked about her sister, who almost a year ago had left home on her 16th birthday: 'She left me a note saying one day we would be together again and I was to write to her. I have a phone number where I can get a message to her.'

'Does she go home for holidays?'

'No.'

Our eyes met. Her definitive no and my response to seeing Carl were all that was needed for us to understand each other. That week, we came up with a plan which would allow us to spend more time together – pairing up pupils who are good at different subjects and can help each other with their homework. 'It's been done in a few schools,' she told me. 'For it to work, we will need the teachers' support.' My best subjects were French and English, hers were Maths and Chemistry, which meant we would be obvious choices to pair together. 'It means we either have to stay late at school, or go to each other's houses. Our parents won't disagree with the head, will they? I'm going to talk to Mr Davis and if he likes the idea, he'll get the others to agree.'

I don't know how she managed it, but all our teachers were enthusiastic and so too were the other pupils. Between all of them the class was sorted out into pairs, a list was printed and a copy given to us all. Carl was hardly pleased about that, said it would have been better if I had waited until my room was finished.

What, another three years?

He then agreed, very reluctantly, that we could use the kitchen.

'I'd rather you stayed in your own home, Emily.'

Where you can keep an eye on us, you mean.

All throughout our senior school years, those joint evenings which progressed to studying in the library and treating ourselves to a coffee out were what kept Marion and I going as we progressed through our teens. My Maths improved – not only did I get every answer correct, but thanks to Marion's tutoring, in most cases I could show the workings-out too. In her case she learnt to speak French, began to enjoy English Literature classes and came first in Maths.

* * *

Unlike me, Marion knew what she wanted to be once she had finished her education. She was going to study Law, she told me. And during our school years, she never once changed her mind.

'And you?' she asked several times over the years. 'With your skill in languages, you could be a translator, travel, all sorts.'

'I want to go to university, I know that,' was my answer, for in a way I had not thought past that.

'One that's a long way from here?' she asked with a curious glance.

'Yes,' I answered, 'as far away from here as possible.'

It was not until we were in the fourth year that we earnestly planned how we were going to be able to get into uni.

'You need the school to suggest you go to a sixth-form college, especially if you want to do A-level Psychology,' Marion told me. 'You can take all your exams there and then apply for a bursary. All you have to do is make your stepfather think you're looking for a job as soon as you've taken your A-levels – a job nearby, of course.'

'And will you have to keep it quiet from your parents as well?'

'Oh, Mum will be delighted when I leave.'

Chapter 54

It was during my third year after the introduction of the buddy system, as we named it, was put in place that I began to use the school library to study in. It was a good excuse to stay later after school. A tiny piece of freedom that made me feel I was a little more in control of my life.

That year was also the one when Gran died. It was not Mum who broke the news to me, but Dad. Funnily enough, when I had heard my mother speaking to him on the phone, my curiosity had been aroused. For once it seemed their conversation was a friendly one, which pleased me as no child really likes their parents to be at loggerheads, do they? On this particular call there were no snappy remarks, instead I heard her saying that yes, she would be grateful, and yes, she would find it difficult, then finally, 'Thank you, Ted' – three words I had never heard her say to him before.

No doubt I would be able to worm out of Dad exactly what they were talking about, for I was very puzzled.

Even though those red-rimmed eyes of hers told me something was wrong, I was pretty sure it didn't have anything to do with me. But by then I had grown used to her outbreaks of depression. Without asking her if she was

OK, a question I had learnt never to pose, I just told her if she needed a break from the boys, I would make her a cup of tea and then take over spooning food into my brothers' mouths – an offer she accepted gratefully.

'Your dad's coming to fetch you from school today,' she told me just as I was leaving. I wanted to ask why, as it was a weekday and I would have homework to do, but as I turned around and saw that she was very close to tears again, the question died in my mouth. *I'll find out later*, I told myself and carried on walking to the bus stop. Not that it prevented me from having a niggling feeling of apprehension all day.

* * *

I can remember what happened after school. Dad was waiting for me outside the gates, it was a sunny afternoon, but I have no recollection of where we went, only what it was he had to tell me. Though I do have a faded picture of him in my head – him leaning across a cafe table and placing his hand on mine and I can almost hear his voice as he gently told me that Gran had died in her sleep.

'A heart attack, she would not have felt anything,' he told me reassuringly.

Numb with shock and grief, I don't think I even cried then – that came later.

Ever since we had moved just over four years ago, I had harboured a dream that once I was free of those mental shackles that Carl had hung on me, she would come back into my life – not just her, but the whole family. Then I would be able to go back to my old life. Now I had to face the reality: it was not going to happen. I would never see her kindly face wreathed in smiles again the moment I entered her house. Even worse was the picture imprinted in my mind of the last time we had seen each other. Her waiting patiently at the gates at the back of the school, her hand outstretched to me. When I had screamed out the word no, I got my last glimpse of Gran looking so desperately sad before I turned and ran away.

I knew how much she had loved both my mother and me – she must have been devastated when we disappeared. I believed then, as I sat opposite my father, that she must have died of a broken heart. Had she hoped as I did that we would walk back into her life? But one day that hope must have died and once hope left her, maybe she saw little reason to remain alive.

This belief was further strengthened when Dad admitted that my mother was not even going to the funeral, but he was.

And not me either? A question I already knew the answer to.

He looked uncomfortable as he searched for the right words to let me down lightly.

'No one blames you for what happened, Emily. You were only nine when your mum and Carl decided to move away. There was nothing you could have done,' he told me.

But there was, wasn't there? I could have told them the truth. A truth I had now left too late to tell.

'They know who's responsible for you being separated from them. Now, I'll tell you something that might make you feel a little better. Your gran certainly did not blame either your mother or you, and she never stopped loving you. She invited me over regularly – she wanted me to tell her as much about you as I could, how you were getting on at school and if you looked well and happy. In fact, every detail I could think of, she wanted to hear. She was so pleased when I told her you were in the A stream. Does that make you feel a little better?'

It didn't, not when I pictured her sitting with Dad, asking all those questions because she missed me so much.

'But now would not be a good time for you to see them again, not after all this time. Let's face it, Carl wouldn't want you to go – you know that. And the last person any of them want to have any contact with is him.'

No matter how Dad tried to camouflage why I was not going by mentioning Carl, this was not the message that registered in my mind: they do blame me for her death. And however much I tried to rationalise the situation when I was older, it is still a belief that has not completely left me.

* * *

The next few weeks were unbearably painful. Mum was also beside herself with guilt and sorrow, while Carl made it clear he didn't want to hear a word about Gran's death.

'She was an old woman, Betty, and old people die. That's normal, so stop wallowing in self-pity!' he told her.

That was the limit of his empathy.

Dear Journal

I'm sorry I have not written to you this week. I'm just so sad that I will never see Gran again. Dad said she never blamed me for what happened, but I do. I never stopped loving her either. But she didn't know that, did she? I expect she thought I had forgotten all about her, but I hadn't. I can't wait till I can leave this place. I try hard not to love my brothers too much because one day I will not to be able to see them again, either.

I made sure I showed as little reaction to Gran's death when Carl was around as possible. Tears had to wait until I was in my room again.

Let him think I don't care, I thought. *That will annoy him more. Concentrate on your schoolwork. Remember, getting to university will be your road to freedom.*

And I knew it was a road I must not waste any time getting on.

Chapter 55

Over the next two years there were a few changes in my life. The first was that Lily decided she did not want me sleeping over anymore. After she caught Paul trying to kiss me, she felt that we were getting too close. I was laughing at his attempt, but it was enough for her to put her foot down. Visit, yes, but better not to sleep over, was what she had told my dad.

And he agreed, which was a few more points lost.

Dad did one thing that was right though – he told me that when the time came, he would help with my applications to go to university. I had told him that Mum and Carl were reluctant for me to go to one too far from home. I don't think he believed that was the only reason I didn't want them to learn what my plans were, it was pretty obvious that I didn't want them to find out until it was too late to stop me.

'I have joint custody of you, not Carl,' he told me. 'Didn't you realise that?'

The answer was no. And in a way, why would I think that? True, I saw him every other weekend, but not staying over at weekends had placed another void in my life.

Yes, we went out for coffee and we talked then, but I had always known he loved Lily and Crystal more than me.

'Joint custody with your mother, not him,' he said firmly. 'All correspondence to do with your further education can start going through me so get yourself into that sixth-form college then I'll notify them that your reports are to be sent to me and anything else to do with your education. Carl can just back off. Don't you worry, just concentrate on your exams and then we'll take it from there.'

And that was a big problem solved.

Well, not quite, as I was to find out.

* * *

Carl accepted me going to sixth-form college and he had also kept his promise and arranged for me to have a holiday job, which would be just Saturdays in term time. It was in a bakery owned by a pleasant man called Colin, who was one of his friends. Naturally, my stepfather insisted I came straight home once the bakery shut, so any socialising with the other staff was out of the question. Still, I enjoyed being away from the house and having a little money of my own. It meant Marion and I could treat ourselves to our cups of coffee and the occasional piece of cake after we had finished studying.

Thank goodness that she and I had a list of homework we had to do jointly. That gave me a break from the oppressive atmosphere in the house as well.

What I had not taken into consideration was the plans that Carl had for me.

* * *

'Colin and his wife are very impressed with your work at the bakery,' my stepfather told me one evening when I had just got in. 'Don't know if they told you, but they're hoping to open up another shop, a bit more upmarket, where they will do afternoon teas and lunches. Colin thinks that you could help run that. What do you think?'

The last thing I want to do.

'That's very nice of him.'

Now try and put him off that idea for the moment, said Reason.

'Have to finish O-levels and get into college for A-levels before I can think straight about working,' I told him, hoping the subject would change.

I understood, or so I thought, why he wanted me to work for his friend – he would know my every movement, who I was friendly with and if I came straight home from work. Another assumption that I was only half-right about. It was the second part of his plan which sent shivers down my spine and made what he really wanted frighteningly clear.

Once all my education was complete, which would not be too long in his mind, Carl wanted me to have his child.

'I've not forgotten you told me you wanted children when you were older. And you're older now, aren't you? You did say that, didn't you?'

Yes, but I don't want yours.

'But what about Mum?'

'Oh, she knows. She doesn't want any more, anyhow.'

It was then that I knew he had just been biding his time until he could legally impregnate me. More than once he had told me that I was the reason he had married my mother. Not that I had believed him then, but I was beginning to now and it scared me.

Well, if you fancy molesting little girls, that's what you do. Find a single mum and there you go!

That's what I had thought ever since I was old enough to realise that I was actually being sexually abused. If I hadn't already known that time was running out for me, I did then. Ignoring the baby bit, I put my head down and tried to look embarrassed.

'Thanks for talking to Colin,' I said. 'He's a really nice man.'

A statement I was beginning to have my doubts about. Just what did my stepdad and his friends all have in common?

'I know he thinks that eventually you would make a good manager. And if you needed a bit of time off' – and here, he flashed me a lascivious smile – 'it wouldn't be a problem, if you get what I mean. So, what do you think of that?'

Help!

'Well, I've got to get all those exams out of the way, haven't I? But tell you what, I'll have a chat with him after work on Saturday.'

Chapter 56

One of the questions I've often heard asked is when someone escapes from their old life and creates a new one, can they really put their past behind them? On the face of it, yes, we can. Or should I say the persona we show to the world tells them that of course we have. Inside our heads though, it's a different matter. The dark shadows of those memories cling on (to the tangle) in our minds as they nibble away the parts that matter, like confidence and self-esteem. That's something I find hard to share with another person. Even when that someone is close to me, the words won't come. For it hurts them to know that with all the love they have given me, I still struggle to put my past life behind me. But that doesn't stop the need to get those thoughts out there. So, what do I do instead of confiding in a human? I do what I've done ever since I was a child – I write those feelings down in my secret journal:

Today, I hurt my head badly. I have a mild concussion, all the symptoms are there. 'You need to get that checked out,' Patrick told me. But I refused to go to the hospital or even to the doctor. Why? I don't like to bother people. Not

that he was going to put up with my refusal. My saying it
was not important just didn't work. There I was, dizzy, with
blurred vision, a blinding headache, feeling nauseous, and
to his annoyance refusing to make sure I was all right. He
told me bluntly that it was not OK to have no concern for
my own health.

Once he had put his foot down, then driven me to
Casualty and back home again, I had to ask myself why
I had been so difficult. Though I knew the answer, didn't
I? My idea of myself is so low, I don't feel worthy of any-
one's time. My partner, although he has tried his best, has
not succeeded in ridding me of those deeply imbedded
thoughts. And this is a very sad reality, one that hit me
hard today.

Good thing you got rid of Fear, said Reason, *now it's*
just me left. You know what you have to do: open that
drawer labelled 'Last Time I saw Carl'. That should make
you believe what you have managed to achieve. Then
when you have done that, get rid of all those negative
thoughts of yours!

I knew that made sense and before I could push that
compunction aside, the drawer slid open.

The last time I saw Carl he had just found out that I had
every intention of going to university. I knew that he had
phoned the college, asking for the results of my exams. And
what had they told him? That they had been sent to my
biological father. Luckily, he was also unaware that as my
mother had joint custody, she would also have been sent a
copy. And she would have been, had I not given the college
Dad's address as my main residence.

If Mum guessed what I had done, she kept quiet – I'm sure that Carl's wanting me to have his child had been enough to turn her into my ally.

* * *

I was called into the Principal's office about my deception. She actually started the interview by asking if everything was all right at home because judging by Carl's bad temper and rudeness when he had shouted down the phone at her assistant, she completely understood why I had kept him in the dark. She reassured me as much as she could that all he had been told was that everything to do with my education had been sent to my biological father. And her assistant, who had the misfortune to take the call, had refused to give him any more information.

'Does he know that I've applied to go to university?'

'No, but he did ask if you were working hard because you still want to go. And he was told that's what sixth-form college is all about – achieving excellent results and gaining the grades for university entry.'

So, he doesn't know everything, I thought gratefully, trying to ignore those worrying niggles that he had found out more than I ever wanted him to know. But I dreaded to think what his temper would be like if he had discovered the whole truth.

For once Carl's rages, which were worst when he was thwarted, had worked in my favour. I can just imagine how he must have ranted and raved at the lack of information being given to him. I only told Miss Evans the Principal that he was against me going to university. Whether she believed that was the only reason I had been so secretive, I don't know. But she reassured me that he was not going to learn any more about my plans from them and I can't tell you how much of a relief that was. Another thing that worked in my favour was that my stepfather would never have credited me with the ability to be deceitful, but then I was fighting for my future while he was trying to prevent me from having one.

Marion and I put our heads together over this latest act of deceit. We had both easily been accepted into the sixth-form college and because our O-level grades were so high, we were given the opportunity to be fast-tracked. Which meant we could take our A-levels in one year instead of two.

'Don't tell him that,' my friend cautioned. 'He'll think you'll be at home for those two years. You can apply for universities without him having a clue and then just scarper.

'Your real dad will help you there, won't he?'

This was one of the rare times she brought his name up as she usually didn't ask questions about my home life. She had a pretty shrewd idea of what it was like, as I had about hers. The two of us shared a joint aim, which did not include complaining about our lives. Instead, we were determined to be positive, to focus on our education and prepare to gain our independence, whichever way we could. If that meant deceiving our families, so be it.

So, Carl had no idea that I had already applied and been interviewed by my university of choice when he made that phone call. I can just imagine what a slap in the face it was for him when the college refused to give him any information. OK, he had managed to wheedle out the fact that I was still aiming to go to uni, but that was all.

Another piece of luck for me was that he did not understand how the further education system worked. For a man who believed that he knew so much, it was surprising he knew so little. Like the issue of releasing information in a joint custody situation. And best of all, he had no idea that A-levels could be fast-tracked and completed in one year instead of two. But still, there was one more worry that refused to go away – that he now knew that it was unlikely that a career running a bakery shop was of any interest to me. That was something he would certainly tackle me about. Still, forewarned was forearmed and I was able to work out a few excuses that I could use when challenged. Not that I was completely confident that they would placate an angry and erratic Carl – Psychology A-level had taught me enough to realise that he was even more unpredictable and irrational when he felt thwarted.

* * *

As a smouldering fire maintains its intense heat when banked down with the dust-like remnants of coal but shows no flames, so Carl's simmering rage was hidden from sight. He was waiting for my term to end before he would allow himself to add enough fuel to turn it into a roaring blaze. He wanted to catch me on the hop, let me keep asking myself the question: had he heard that snippet of information or not?

He waited until the day he believed was my last day at college before the summer holidays – which it was. This was also the day that Marion and I were told by the Principal that because of her report and our expected results, we had obtained unconditional university places. Mine was at a northern red brick to read English and French, while Marion was going to LSE to study Law.

Once I had that knowledge tucked away in my mind, all I wanted was to get through the summer, work as many days as I could at the bakery and save up some money. I felt a bit guilty about not being able to tell Colin the truth, but I had no choice but to let him continue hoping I would end up working full-time for him. I just hoped that Carl had not put two and two together and worked out that this was never going to be my intention.

He had.

As soon as I walked into the house and saw his grim expression, I knew. I just prayed that I could somehow defuse his anger. But I didn't have long to put that to the test, because even before I had taken my things through to my room, his bombardment of questions started to fly at me.

'So, Emily, what are your plans for the holidays?' was the first seemingly innocuous one.

I told him that I was going to be working at the bakery most days.

'And you have talked to Colin, have you, about working full-time for him next year?'

'Yes,' I said, keeping my fingers crossed that my answer would satisfy him.

It didn't – the smirk that appeared on his face told me that.

'So' – and here, he held my gaze – 'you're still leading my mate up the garden path, are you? You've no intention of working for him, have you?'

I tried to bypass that question by saying I had to wait for the results of my exams before I could make any plans.

An answer he made clear that he did not believe.

'Come off it! Do you think I was born yesterday? You're planning on at least another four years of studying so don't lie to me and say you aren't.'

Before I could think of anything to say to that, he told me in a deceptively calm voice that he was disappointed I had not confided in him, if that was what I wanted. However calm he might sound, I could sense him stoking his rage with every question and remark he threw at me though.

'I expect your dad knows all about your plans, doesn't he? But you didn't think I was good enough to be told, did you?'

I tried to pluck some placating words out of thin air, but Carl, sensing my hesitation, just gave me a scornful look.

'Oh, don't waste your breath trying to palm me off with some excuse or other! There's no point talking any longer, is there? Now do me a favour and go out to my car – there's a bag in the boot I want brought in.'

Surely that's not all he's going to say to me, I thought, wondering just what was in that bag that he wanted me to fetch. I wouldn't have put it past him to have brought home some bondage gear or a new sex toy, for the pornography he showed me was getting weirder and his sexual advances had become more adventurous and disgusting. If so, he would enjoy imagining me quaking with fear as I waited with him watching me until it was time for Mum and the boys to go to bed.

My brothers might have heard him ridiculing me and even watched wide-eyed as he pulled up my jumper in front of them, trapping my arms, and undid my bra before grabbing hold of one of my exposed breasts. They saw it as a game, which of course it was to him – a very sick one. But he was careful, apart from the odd slap across my face, not to show them his violent side.

'OK, what am I looking for?' I asked, scarcely believing that I was being let off the hook so lightly.

'A bag of shopping, that's all,' he told me, tossing a bunch of keys in my direction.

Out of the corner of my eye I saw my mother's face turn a chalky white as she stood up and I heard her utter his name as I went outside – I still had no idea what her reaction was all about.

Opening the deep boot of his car, I saw a bag tucked in the very far corner. As I leant into it, my arm outstretched to reach the bag, I suddenly had a flash of realisation and knew why he had sent me out to get it.

He had moved so fast to follow me that before I had a chance to straighten up, his knee was rammed onto my back, pinning me in place as his hands gripped my shoulders to prevent me moving.

'You two-faced little bitch!' he hissed. 'You and your dad have plotted this together, haven't you? You think I'm going to let you swan off after everything I've done for you? Well, there's only one way you're going to be leaving here . . .'

I felt one hand release me and stretch upwards towards the lid of the boot.

I then heard a blood-curdling scream coming from my mother as she hurled herself against us, breaking his grip on me. Just as the lid crashed downwards where my head had been, I flew sideways. My mother's intervention meant I only received a glancing blow to the side of my head.

I could feel the blood trickling down my face and into my eyes.

Through ringing ears, I could hear my mother shouting, 'So what are you thinking of doing, Carl, killing us all? She's not worth it! Think of your sons being without a father. Now go, just go and don't you dare come back tonight or I'm warning you, I'll call the police!'

I'm sure she said a lot more than that, but I was only half-conscious and totally in shock. Whatever else she might have said to him, it was enough for him to jump in the car and drive off at high speed.

For the second time, my mother had to help me up. Sick and dizzy, I leant on her as she slowly led me into the house. All I wanted was to lie down and close my eyes.

'Not until I'm sure you don't have concussion,' she told me, her voice full of concern.

If I had felt a bit better, I might have asked what she thought someone who has just had a hard blow to the side of the head and lost consciousness had.

Mum examined the cut and bathed it in antiseptic to make sure it was clean. It wasn't deep and didn't need stitches, she proclaimed. She made me some sweet caffeine-free herbal tea, before giving me her arm again and leading me into my room.

* * *

I should have fallen into a deep sleep straight away, but all the questions churning in my mind kept me awake.

Would Carl, the man who had given me a silver chain and told me he saw me as his daughter, really have crashed that heavy boot down on my head? Was it my skull he had wanted to shatter?

Or did he want to drive it into my face and tear my skin until the bones were exposed?

Did he want to scar me for life so no one else would want me?

And what excuse would he have used to the people who would question him? Would he convince them that it was just a dreadful accident?

And to himself, how could he justify that act?

That I had driven him to it, that he had no choice?

Could he really have lived with that?

I just couldn't get my throbbing head around these questions. They kept repeating themselves until finally I fell into a deep, but troubled sleep.

When I woke, it was light – I must have slept for hours, I realised.

I hardly had the energy to move, but move I must; first to the bathroom and then to the phone. I couldn't stay here any longer, I knew that. Mum had got the better of him this time, but what about the next time it happened?

He might return home all charming and pleasant, he might even tell me he was just trying to scare me and that he was sorry, or he could return full of the confidence of a man who believed he was justified in his actions. There was just no telling with him – he was completely unpredictable. The one thing I was really afraid of was believing I would be at home for another year, he would stop at nothing to impregnate me.

A bulging stomach would keep me tied to him, wouldn't it?

By covering my bed with several books, and using the word 'homework', which in fact I did not have, I had already managed to prevent him from coming into my bed several times. I doubted if those excuses would work now.

After everything he had done to me from when I was a small child to just the day before, I doubted he would have had any compunction about adding rape to his list of depravities. I knew too that however much I struggled, he would overpower me. And however much I screamed and begged for help, would anyone come to my aid? And did my mother care enough to intervene a second time?

As soon as I was able, I crept out of bed and took myself into the room where the phone was. Mum was already up, looking even more haggard than she had the day before. I doubt she had managed to have a dreamless sleep either. Without saying anything, I picked up the phone and dialled Dad's number.

'I need to get out of here,' was all I said.

The only question he asked was, 'Is he there?' When I answered him with a short no, he just told me to pack what I needed and to give him an hour to get to me.

I told Mum I wanted to say goodbye to my brothers before I left. If I was looking for any show of emotion at this point then none came, she just said, 'All right.' I then went into my room and threw haphazardly as much as I could into a selection of carrier bags, which Mum handed to me wordlessly.

Was she sad I was leaving? I certainly know that there was a lump in my throat. Whatever sins she had committed, she was still my mother. Did I hope there would be a final hug, that she would tell me I would be missed, and even more important, that she was sorry, so sorry she had stood by and watched what was happening but never once tried to put a stop to it? Surely she must have known that as soon as I walked out of the door, she was unlikely to see me again. This was her final chance to say it. Or was it a relief that I was actually going?

Even now I still don't know what her feelings were – she never told me.

Unlike my brothers, her face gave little away, but the boys burst into tears when I said my goodbyes.

'When are you coming back?' they asked.

The one question I didn't want to answer, for I had little intention of ever returning.

'I'll send you lots of postcards,' I told them. 'You'll be able to take them to school and show your friends.'

A promise that diverted them from asking me again when I would return so maybe their tears ceased because they thought I really would.

When I hugged them both, I felt such a pang of grief. I might not have wanted to love my brothers, because from the moment they came into the world, I knew that one day I would want to leave. But I had found it impossible not to feel a deep affection for them. Just six and seven years old, I was going to miss them so much. My arms wrapped around them in those last hugs. None of the reasons I was leaving were their faults, were they? They might have Carl's genes, but perhaps those of my mother were stronger, for they reminded me of my cousins when we had all been small.

Before they could ask any more questions, I heard the sound of Dad's car pulling up.

Mum actually helped me carry out all those bags.

I thought I would try just once to make her see sense: 'Mum, why won't you leave him?' I asked. 'You've not been happy for years.'

'And where would I go?' she said wearily.

Our eyes met and there was the flicker of remorse that I had seen all those years ago. She must have felt that by giving in to Carl, she had burnt all her bridges with her own family. They must have been so angry with her for hurting Gran. She had not even gone to the funeral. Probably too afraid, I had thought then. But who else would understand, if she did not tell them?

'You could let your sisters know the truth . . .'

She looked at me then with a slightly sardonic smile on her face.

'I don't think I could do that, Emily. Now do you?'

That was the closest she ever got to admitting how much in the wrong she had been over all those years. The fact that I was finally escaping was what gave me the ability to forgive her – I might no longer have any love left for her, nor wish to receive any in return, but still I felt something which made me want to reassure her that my life was not completely ruined.

'I have a place at university,' I told her.

'I know, Emily, you were fast-tracked. You forget I have joint custody as well.'

She had kept my secret after all.

'So, are you going to stay with him?'

'You don't understand, Emily. I still love him. Now go!'

That was the last conversation we ever had.

* * *

Once in the car, I didn't turn to look back at the forlorn woman holding the hands of two tear-streaked little boys.

I looked straight ahead.

I think it was the phone call my father had been waiting to receive ever since Gran had shared her fears with him. He placed a hand gently on my shoulder, smiled as I turned to him and said, 'Let's get you back to mine.' To my relief, he didn't ask any questions during that drive.

You can leave now, I told Fear, and without a murmur of protest, it moved out of the space that it had occupied since I was four.

It had a new home to go to, hadn't it?

Epilogue

June 2006

Dear Journal

I can write to you in English now! I'm free, I can stay with Dad until I go to uni!

Surprise, surprise, Lily found me a job in a coffee shop! But what did she do first? Pulled out all my clothes and tossed them in a black sack. 'Oxfam for those,' she said. 'Maybe there's a nun running away from a convent who might want them.'

She had a point.

'Shopping is needed,' she told me. 'Your dad's given me his credit card. Time you looked like a teenager, an attractive one.'

Lily being friendly, well, that's a first! She did tell me that the reason she hadn't wanted me sleeping over was that Paul had such a crush on me. And she knew (a) I wasn't interested and (b) I would leave one day. Anyhow, he has a girlfriend now, so problem solved.

She took me to Gap. Now that's a shop Carl would never have let me go to. She made me say yes to a pair of straight-legged blue jeans, some really bright coloured T-shirts and even a pair of leggings. All my shoes were chucked out as well. Now I've got strappy sandals and a pair of boots with heels that were in the sale. And you should see my make-up!

I can't believe how different I feel.

Lily says I look trendy.

What, me?

September 2006

Hello again, Journal

I just love being at uni! I've made some friends already – they invited me to a party and I can't believe what a great time I had.

I didn't tell them it was my first one! And they didn't guess. They are all so cool. None of them mind about me sorting my veg into different colours – they think it makes me more interesting!

Spoke to Marion on the phone and she's happy too. Says London is super cool! She wants us to meet up later this year.

That will be so good.

February 2009

Dear Journal

I met someone last night. I was in the bar where we all hang out and I looked up and how romantic! It's such a cliché, I know, but our eyes did meet. His are a beautiful deep green. I thought he was just drop-dead gorgeous, he told me he thought I was! Well, he did after he bought me a couple of drinks.

We talked and talked, I just didn't want the evening to end. He's a third-year student like me, only he's studying science. And guess what? He's asked to see me tomorrow. Can't wait!

His name is Patrick and I just know he's special.

October 2009

Amazing, I never thought this could happen! I've moved in with Patrick – but not until I opened up and told him everything.

He wrapped his arms around me and held me close. Told me he would keep me safe. That I have a new life now and so many people like me. All he wants is for me to feel cared for.

Didn't I say he was special? He really is. I can't believe my luck that I found him.

September 2010

Here we are with our degrees, not just any degree but an honours one.

And you know what I'm going to do?

When I get my certificate, I'm going to send a copy of it to Carl and sign it from the idiot savant.

Petty, you might think.

Maybe, but I'll tell you one thing, that cloak of inferiority that he had draped around my shoulders for all those years – well, it's going with it!

I'm posting it in London when I meet up with Marion.

Let him think that's where I live.

May 2012

Hello, Journal!

Guess what? We've moved to Ireland, to County Cork – Patrick was missing it so much. Oh, did I not tell you, that's where he's from?

We've found a lovely cottage to live in. It's in a small village and the people here are just so friendly. It will be a great place to bring up children and yes, we are planning that.

We've only been here a week and Patrick says I'm already sounding Irish. And yes, it does rain a lot, but then it makes everything so green.

That's why it's called the Emerald Isle, isn't it?

January 2019

Dear Journal

OK, you know there are times when I have the wobbles. Can't escape the past all the time. But then who can? And as for that nasty little demon Fear, it has a knack of paying me the odd uninvited visit.

It's a good thing I have you to write in. Because once I have, I can find the strength to shove it away as hard as I can. Oh, it mutters away for a bit and then it disappears.

June 2020

Dear Journal

Today, I had my first scan, watched that little tadpole wriggling away. My third baby! And guess what? He or she is due to arrive at Christmas.

Sonia might think Santa brought the baby! So, I take her hand, place it on my stomach and watch her eyes grow *huge as I explain that's where babies grow. I can't wait to see her face once she can feel those tiny feet kicking away.*

None of us can wait till this Christmas.

And here's a selfish thought – guess who will have to do the housework this year!

Went maternity clothes shopping. Can you believe all the clothes were in navy blue and dark burgundy! No way! Eventually I found what I wanted in a pretty pale yellow and another in a lovely deep pink.

Perfect for Christmas!

Acknowledgements

This book has been a labour of love and tears. Being fully open about my life has been one of the hardest, yet fulfilling experiences of my life. I would have never imagined myself writing acknowledgements for a book about my past – up until a certain age, I didn't think I'd be alive. Some people have saved me; they didn't know it, but they pulled me out from the darkest hole possible.

To my partner, you have seen it all, you witnessed the tears, the fears, the years of therapy. You remained by my side through it all. You showed me what love truly means. I always said even if one day we part ways, I'll love you forever and be grateful for all you have given me. For the first time ever, I didn't feel like a burden, an inconvenience, I felt alive.

To my children, my girls, the loves of my life, what can I even say? You are everything, you both simply are. Your smiles, laughs, cuddles and kisses, they're the reason to wake up in the morning. I've been called a lot of names, but 'Mummy' is, and always will be, my favourite. I look at you two and cannot believe I made you, *me*! You are all I wish I was, so brave, smart, hilarious, strong-headed, kind and beyond gorgeous. I'm amazed every time I look into your eyes. I hope one day when you are older and start having questions, you will read this book. I hope you will be proud of me.

To my baby, as I'm writing this, you are happily kicking in my belly. Know that you are so loved already. You sure do challenge me already, but I cannot wait to meet you and show you our beautiful family.

To Toni, it's so strange how sometimes people who haven't been in your life long can make a huge impact. You are just that. I never thought anyone would be interested in hearing about my life. Not only were you interested, but you made me feel less alone. For the first time I had a voice worth hearing. Your kindness is beyond belief, you've been like a surrogate mum. You never judged me, I always felt comfortable telling you the worst details, those that still bring me shame. You gave me hope.

To my dear readers, thank you for your support, thank you for listening to my story. My biggest wish is for it to bring a glimmer of hope to those still suffering. You are not alone, far from it. I wanted to share my darkest moments with you because I know a lot of you will relate, perhaps for the first time. I want you all to know that things *will* get better, you don't have to suffer in silence. Keep safe, everyone.

Childline

You can talk to Childline about anything. No problem is too big or too small. Call free on 0800 1111.

Childline is a UK charity supporting young people in the UK, and there is also Child Helpline International for organisations in other countries that may be able to help. For more information, visit www.childline.org.uk.